AF782007

CHILDREN'S ISSUES, LAWS AND PROGRAMS

MEDICATING FOSTER CARE CHILDREN WITH PSYCHOTROPIC DRUGS

AN EXAMIMATION

CHILDREN'S ISSUES, LAWS AND PROGRAMS

Additional books in this series can be found on Nova's website under the Series tab.

Additional E-books in this series can be found on Nova's website under the E-books tab.

SOCIAL ISSUES, JUSTICE AND STATUS

Additional books in this series can be found on Nova's website under the Series tab.

Additional E-books in this series can be found on Nova's website under the E-books tab.

CHILDREN'S ISSUES, LAWS AND PROGRAMS

MEDICATING FOSTER CARE CHILDREN WITH PSYCHOTROPIC DRUGS

AN EXAMIMATION

ROBERT L. RAY
AND
MACKENZIE A. WATKINS
EDITORS

Nova Science Publishers, Inc.
New York

For permission to use material from this book please contact us:
Telephone 631-231-7269; Fax 631-231-8175
Web Site: http://www.novapublishers.com

LIBRARY OF CONGRESS CATALOGING-IN-PUBLICATION DATA

ISBN 978-1-61942-889-8

Published by Nova Science Publishers, Inc. † New York

CONTENTS

PREFACE

Foster children, often being removed from neglectful or abusive homes, are one of the country's most vulnerable populations. With the often traumatic circumstances that define their early lives, it is no wonder studies show their tendency for more mental health conditions than other children. Facing these and other significant challenges surrounding foster care programs, state authorities, caseworkers, and parents, are given few options on appropriate treatments. These options often include prescribing heavy-duty psychotropic drugs such as antidepressants and, in some cases, even antipsychotics - drugs which have little research available supporting their use in children. This book examines the practice of medicating America's foster children with a focus on the financial and societal costs.

Chapter 1- Foster children have often been removed from abusive or neglectful homes and tend to have more mental health conditions than other children. Treatment of these conditions may include psychotropic drugs, but the risks these drugs pose specifically to children are not well understood. Medicaid, which is administered by states and overseen by the Department of Health and Human Services (HHS), provides prescription drug coverage to foster children.

For selected states, GAO examined (1) 2008 rates of psychotropic prescriptions for foster and nonfoster children and (2) state oversight of psychotropic prescriptions for foster children through October 2011. GAO selected Florida, Maryland, Massachusetts, Michigan, Oregon, and Texas primarily for geographic diversity and size of the foster care population, and analyzed state Medicaid fee-forservice and foster care data from selected states for 2008. 2008 was the most recent year of prescription data available at the start of the audit. Maryland's 2008 foster care data were unreliable and could not be analyzed. GAO contracted with expert child psychiatrists to provide a clinical perspective on our methodology and analysis, reviewed regulations and state policies, and interviewed federal and state officials. Results cannot be generalized to other states.

Chapter 2- Foster children, often being removed from neglectful or abusive homes, are one of the country's most vulnerable populations. With the often traumatic circumstances that define their early lives, it is no wonder studies show their tendency for more mental health conditions than other children. Facing these and other significant challenges surrounding foster care programs, state authorities, caseworkers, and parents, are given few options on appropriate treatments. As our witnesses will discuss today, these options often include prescribing heavy-duty psychotropic drugs such as antidepressants and, in some cases, even antipsychotics – drugs which have little research available supporting their use in children.

Chapter 3- Chairman Carper, Ranking Member Brown, and members of the subcommittee, thank you for the opportunity to testify before you this morning about the use of psychotropic medications among children in foster care. First, I would like to acknowledge the leadership demonstrated by Congress in this area already, most recently in the reauthorization of title IV-B of the Social Security Act. In September, Congress acted on an administration proposal to provide HHS with additional authority in the Child and Family Services Improvement and Innovations Act of 2011 (Public Law 112-34) to require states to address the trauma needs of children and to develop protocols for monitoring the use of psychotropic drugs among children in foster care. Other notable Congressional work includes the passage of the Fostering Connections to Success and Increasing Adoptions Act, which requires the use of medical homes and oversight of prescription medications for children in foster care, and the recent work of the Senate Caucus on Foster Youth, led by senators Landrieu and Grassley, to highlight the issue of psychotropics. In 2009, the Subcommittee on Income Security and Family Support of the House Committee on Ways and Means held a hearing on prescription psychotropic drug use among children in foster care. Additionally, I would like to thank this Committee for requesting that the Government Accountability Office review the use of psychotropics with children in foster care, as it has produced a comprehensive and useful report that can help guide ongoing action. As I have noted, much work has occurred already, and the hearing today furthers this critical conversation. Together, this work will advance the child welfare and mental health fields and truly benefit some of the most vulnerable children in our society.

Chapter 4- Medicaid is the nation's health care safety net. Jointly financed by the states and the federal government, Medicaid will spend more than $400 billion this year to provide health care to more than 60 million Americans. The program is administered by the states within a broad federal framework which leads to enormous variation across states in terms of who is covered, what services are provided, and how those services are delivered and paid for. Furthermore, within any given state, Medicaid's role is broad, varied, and complex. Medicaid funds more than 40 percent of all births, and the majority of all publicly financed long-term care in this country. It also provides most of the nation's funding for HIV/AIDS-related treatments, mental health services, and others. It is therefore very difficult to talk simplistically about Medicaid (either nationally, or within a state), despite its incredible importance in the U.S. health care system.

Chapter 5- I am a child psychiatrist at Seattle Children's Hospital, a professor at the University of Washington, and the medical director of Child Study and Treatment Center, the State psychiatric hospital for youth in Washington State.

The high risk practices identified by the GAO study raise significant concerns regarding the treatment of severely mentally ill and vulnerable youth. Although the focus of this study is on foster care, the concerns raised are relevant to all children and adolescents prescribed psychotropic drugs.

Children in foster care often have emotional and behavioral difficulties. The high rate of medication use in this population is not a new discovery, nor does the use of these drugs always imply bad practice. Several psychiatric medications have been studied and approved for use in children and adolescents. When prescribed correctly, these treatments can help reduce suffering and enhance the functioning of young people.

However, it is also well documented that many children in the child welfare system do not receive high quality psychiatric services. Treatment too often occurs during times of crisis, without adequate support or access to skilled clinicians and programs capable of providing effective social and behavioral interventions.

In: Medicating Foster Care Children...
Editors: R. L. Ray and M. A. Watkins
ISBN: 978-1- 61942-889-8

Chapter 1

FOSTER CHILDREN: HHS GUIDANCE COULD HELP STATES IMPROVE OVERSIGHT OF PSYCHOTROPIC PRESCRIPTIONS*

United States Government Accountability Office

WHY GAO DID THIS STUDY

Foster children have often been removed from abusive or neglectful homes and tend to have more mental health conditions than other children. Treatment of these conditions may include psychotropic drugs, but the risks these drugs pose specifically to children are not well understood. Medicaid, which is administered by states and overseen by the Department of Health and Human Services (HHS), provides prescription drug coverage to foster children.

For selected states, GAO examined (1) 2008 rates of psychotropic prescriptions for foster and nonfoster children and (2) state oversight of psychotropic prescriptions for foster children through October 2011. GAO selected Florida, Maryland, Massachusetts, Michigan, Oregon, and Texas primarily for geographic diversity and size of the foster care population, and analyzed state Medicaid fee-forservice and foster care data from selected states for 2008.

* This is an edited, reformatted and augmented version of GAO-12-201, a report by GAO to Congressional Requesters, dated December 2011.

2008 was the most recent year of prescription data available at the start of the audit. Maryland's 2008 foster care data were unreliable and could not be analyzed. GAO contracted with expert child psychiatrists to provide a clinical perspective on our methodology and analysis, reviewed regulations and state policies, and interviewed federal and state officials. Results cannot be generalized to other states.

What GAO Recommends

GAO recommends that HHS consider endorsing guidance for states on best practices for overseeing psychotropic prescriptions for foster children. HHS agreed with our recommendation.

What GAO Found

Foster children in the five states GAO analyzed were prescribed psychotropic drugs at higher rates than nonfoster children in Medicaid during 2008. The higher rates do not necessarily indicate inappropriate prescribing practices, but according to research, experts consulted, and certain federal and state officials, could be due in part to foster children's greater mental health needs, greater exposure to traumatic experiences, and the challenges of coordinating their medical care. However, prescriptions to foster children in these states were also more likely to have indicators of potential health risks. According to experts, no evidence supports the concomitant use of five or more psychotropic drugs in adults or children, yet hundreds of both foster and nonfoster children in the five states had such a drug regimen. Similarly, thousands of foster and nonfoster children were prescribed doses higher than the maximum levels cited in guidelines developed by Texas based on FDA-approved labels, which experts said increases the potential for adverse side effects and does not typically increase the efficacy of the drugs to any significant extent. Further, foster and nonfoster children under 1 year old were prescribed psychotropic drugs, which GAO's experts said have no established use for mental health conditions in infants and could result in serious adverse effects.

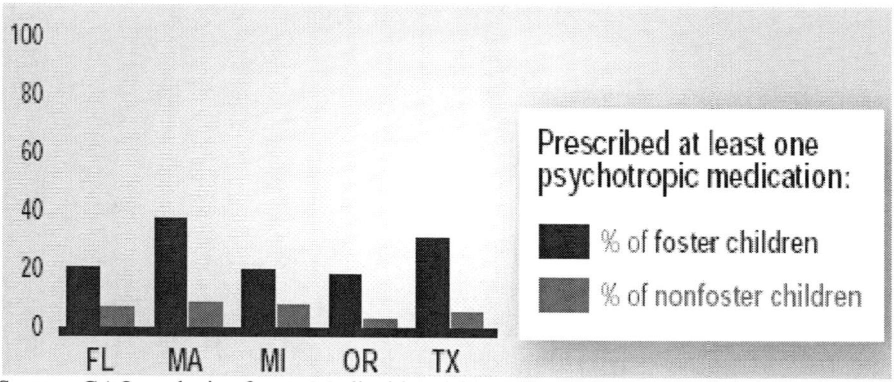

Source: GAO analysis of state Medicaid and foster care data.

Psychotropic Prescription Rates for Foster and Nonfoster Children Age 0-17 in Medicaid Fee-for-Service in Five States.

The six selected states' foster children fall short of best principles guidelines published by the American Academy of Child and Adolescent Psychiatry (AACAP). The guidelines, which states are not required to follow, cover four categories.

- Consent: Each state has some practices consistent with AACAP consent guidelines, such as identifying caregivers empowered to give consent.
- Oversight: Each state has procedures consistent with some but not all oversight guidelines, which include monitoring rates of prescriptions.
- Consultation: Five states have implemented some but not all guidelines, which include providing consultations by child psychiatrists by request.
- Information: Four states have created websites about psychotropic drugs for clinicians, foster parents, and other caregivers.

This variation is expected because states set their own guidelines. HHS has not endorsed specific measures for state oversight of psychotropic prescriptions for foster children. HHS-endorsed guidance could help close gaps in oversight of psychotropic prescriptions and increase protections for these vulnerable children.

ABBREVIATIONS

AACAP	American Academy of Child and Adolescent Psychiatry
ACF	Administration for Children and Families
ADHD	Attention Deficit Hyperactivity Disorder
BPCA	Best Pharmaceuticals for Children Act
CFSR	Child and Family Services Review
CMS	Centers for Medicare & Medicaid Services
CWS	Child Welfare Services
DFPS	Texas Department of Family and Protective Services
FDA	Food and Drug Administration
HHS	Department of Health and Human Services
HMO	Health Maintenance Organization
MCPAP	Massachusetts Child Psychiatry Access Project
MMIS	Medicaid Management Information System
MMPP	Maryland Medicaid Pharmacy Program
NIMH	National Institute of Mental Health
NSCAW	National Survey of Child and Adolescent Well-Being
OBRA	Omnibus Budget Reconciliation Act
PA	Prior Authorization
PREA	Pediatric Research Equity Act
SSRI	Selective Serotonin Reuptake Inhibitors

December 14, 2011
Congressional Requesters

Children placed in foster care are among our nation's most vulnerable populations. Often having been removed from abusive or neglectful homes, they tend to have more numerous and serious medical and mental health conditions than do other children.[1] Treatment of mental illness may include prescribing psychotropic drugs, such as antidepressants and antipsychotics. Because foster children are under state care, they typically receive prescription drugs and other medical services through Medicaid, a joint federal-state program that finances health care coverage for certain low-income populations.[2]

The use of psychotropic drugs has been shown to effectively treat mental disorders, such as attention deficit hyperactivity disorder (ADHD), bipolar disorder, depression, and schizophrenia. While many psychotropic drugs that have been approved by the Food and Drug Administration (FDA) as safe and effective in adults have not been similarly approved for children of all ages, prescribing them to children is legal and common medical practice in many instances. According to the National Institute of Mental Health (NIMH), some children with severe mental health conditions would suffer serious consequences without such medication.[3] However, psychotropic drugs can also have serious side effects in adults, including irreversible movement disorders, seizures, and an increased risk for diabetes over the long term. Further, additional risks these drugs pose specifically to children are not well understood.[4]

States are responsible for running their Medicaid and foster care programs, but the programs are administered at the federal level by the Department of Health and Human Services (HHS) through the Centers for Medicare & Medicaid Services (CMS) and the Administration for Children and Families (ACF), respectively. HHS may issue regulations, provide guidance on some issues, or simply provide informational resources for states to consider for their programs, the latter being the case for psychotropic drugs provided to children in state custody. Among these resources are best principles developed by the American Academy of Child and Adolescent Psychiatry (AACAP), a nonprofit professional association. While HHS does not require states to follow these guidelines, AACAP developed them as a model to help inform state monitoring programs for youth in state custody. AACAP guidelines point out that "as a result of several highly publicized cases of questionable inappropriate prescribing, treating youth in state custody with psychopharmacological agents has come under increasingly intense scrutiny," leading to state implementation of consent, authorization, and monitoring procedures.[5] More recently, Congress enacted the Child and Family Services Improvement and Innovation Act in September 2011, requiring states that apply for certain federal child welfare grants to establish protocols for the appropriate use and monitoring of psychotropic drugs prescribed to foster children.[6]

You requested that we examine psychotropic drugs prescribed to foster children. In this report, for selected states we (1) compared rates of psychotropic drug prescriptions for foster children and nonfoster children covered by Medicaid in 2008, including indicators of potential health risks, and (2) examined federal and state oversight policies in effect for psychotropic drugs prescribed to foster children through October 2011. Our full scope and methodology is provided in appendix I.

To provide a clinical perspective on our methodology and data analysis, we contracted with two child psychiatrists with clinical and research expertise in the use of psychotropic drugs in children. Dr. Jon McClellan is an attending psychiatrist at the Seattle Children's Hospital; a professor at the University of

Washington School of Medicine; and the medical director at Washington's Child Study and Treatment Center, the children psychiatric hospital for the state of Washington. He is board certified in psychiatry and child and adolescent psychiatry. Dr. Michael Naylor is an associate professor at the University of Illinois at Chicago, School of Medicine, and the director of the Behavioral Health and Welfare Program, which was formed to address the mental health needs of the most severely disturbed children in state care. He directs the Clinical Services in Psychopharmacology program, which provides an independent review of all psychotropic medication consent requests for foster children in Illinois. He is board certified in child and adolescent psychiatry, general psychiatry, and sleep disorders medicine.

To compare rates of psychotropic drug prescriptions in foster children and nonfoster children covered by Medicaid, we reviewed calendar year 2008 fee-for-service prescription claims and foster care data for Florida, Maryland, Massachusetts, Michigan, Oregon, and Texas.[7] At the start of our audit, 2008 data were the most recent calendar year prescription claims data available from CMS. These states were selected primarily for geographic diversity and the size of their foster care populations. However, we then excluded Maryland from our analysis due to the unreliability of its foster care data. Because the audit was limited to children in these nonrandomly selected states, the results cannot be generalized to other states or populations. In consultation with our experts, we developed a list of psychotropic drugs likely to be prescribed in the six selected states by reviewing each state's list of approved drugs, and a list of psychotropic drugs published by NIMH. Based on our experts' recommendations, we excluded some drugs likely to be for nonmental health purposes (such as anticonvulsants) from our overall analysis of psychotropic prescription rates, but included them in our analysis of concomitant prescriptions—that is, prescriptions for multiple drugs to be taken concurrently—and our analysis of gaps in medications.[8] As such, we are likely understating the percentage of children prescribed psychotropic drugs for mental health purposes. See appendix III for the listing of psychotropic drugs used in our overall analysis.

To identify prescribed drug regimens that have potential health risk indicators, we, among other things, consulted with our experts, performed literature searches, and reviewed state guidelines. Based on this, our final indicators of potential health risks were: concomitant prescriptions of five or more drugs, prescriptions exceeding dosage guidelines in the Psychotropic Medication Utilization Parameters for Texas Foster Children, and psychotropic prescriptions for children under 1 year old. In addition, we evaluated gaps of 7 to 29 days in prescriptions of a drug to identify non adherence to drug regimens, which can pose significant risks to a patient. Because prescription claims do not include diagnosis data, we were not able to examine the clinical indications used to justify psychotropic prescriptions. Further, prescribers should weigh the benefits and drawbacks of drug regimens on a case-by-case basis. As such, determining the appropriateness of prescriptions without patient-level reviews by medical experts is impossible.

To determine federal and state oversight policies in effect for prescribing psychotropic drugs to foster children through October 2011, we interviewed officials from CMS, ACF, and the six selected states' Medicaid and foster care agencies. We also reviewed policies, statutes, and regulations related to the prescribing of psychotropic drugs to foster children. Based on a literature review and discussions with officials from HHS, we selected AACAP's guidelines as a basis for assessing the extent to which selected states were implementing recommended practices.

We performed this audit from February 2010 through November 2011 in accordance with generally accepted government auditing standards. Those standards require that we plan and perform the audit to obtain sufficient, appropriate evidence to provide a reasonable basis for our findings and conclusions based on our audit objectives. We believe that the evidence obtained provides a reasonable basis for our findings and conclusions based on our audit objectives.

BACKGROUND

Foster care begins when a child is removed from his or her parents or guardians and placed under the responsibility of a state child welfare agency. Removal from the home can occur because of reasons such as physical abuse or neglect. It can also occur when a child's own behavior or condition is beyond the control of his or her family or poses a threat to their community. As we have previously reported, children in foster care exhibit more numerous and serious medical conditions, including mental health conditions, than do other children.[9]

Foster care may be provided by a family member, caregivers previously unknown to the child, or a group home or institution. Ideally, foster care is an intermediate step towards a permanent family home. When reuniting the child with his or her parents or guardian is not in the child's best interest, caseworkers seek a new permanent home for the child, such as an adoptive home or guardianship. However, some children remain in foster care until they reach adulthood.

Psychotropic drugs affect brain activity associated with mental processes and behavior. These drugs are also called psychotherapeutic drugs. While psychotropic drugs can have significant benefits for those with mental illnesses, they can also have side effects ranging from mild to serious. Table 1 highlights the psychotropic drug classes studied in this report and provides examples of drugs within those classes, as well as conditions treated and possible side effects. Specific information about each drug can be found in appendix II.

Foster Children Have Higher Rates of Psychotropic Drug Prescriptions and Indicators of Potential Health Risks

Foster children in each of the five selected states were prescribed psychotropic drugs at higher rates than were nonfoster children in Medicaid during 2008.[10] These states spent over $375 million for prescriptions provided through fee-for-service programs to foster and nonfoster children.[11] The higher rates do not necessarily indicate inappropriate prescribing practices, as they could be due to foster children's greater exposure to traumatic experiences and the unique challenges of coordinating their medical care.[12] However, psychotropic drug claims for foster children were also more likely to show the indicators of potential health risks that we established with our experts. According to our experts, no evidence supports the concomitant use of five or more psychotropic drugs in adults or children, yet hundreds of both foster and nonfoster children were prescribed such a medication regimen. Similarly, thousands of foster and nonfoster children were prescribed doses exceeding maximum levels cited in guidelines based on information in FDA-approved drug labels, which our experts said increases the potential for adverse side effects, and does not typically increase the efficacy of the drugs to any significant extent.[13] Further, foster and nonfoster children under 1 year old were prescribed psychotropic drugs, which our experts said have no established use for mental health conditions in infants and could result in serious adverse effects.

Table 1. Psychotropic Drug Classes

Drug class	Examples of drugs	Types of conditions treated by drug class	Examples of possible adverse side effects
ADHD drugs	Atomoxetine (Strattera) Lisdexamfetamine dimesylate (Vyvanse) Methylphenidate (Ritalin, Concerta) Amphetamine (Adderall) Dextroamphetamine (Dexedrine, Dextrostat)	Attention deficit hyperactivity disorder	Decreased appetite Tics Psychosis
Anti-anxiety	Clonazepam (Klonopin) Lorazepam (Ativan) Alprazolam (Xanax)	Generalized anxiety disorder, Post-traumatic stress dis-order,Social phobias	Dependence Drowsiness and dizziness Blurred vision Nightmares
Anti-depressants	Fluoxetine (Prozac) Citalopram (Celexa) Sertraline (Zoloft) Paroxetine (Paxil) Escitalopram (Lexapro) Venlafaxine (Effexor) Duloxetine (Cymbalta) Bupropion (Wellbutrin)	Depression Generalized anxiety disorder Obsessive-compulsive disorder Social phobia	Suicidal thoughts Sleeplessness or drowsiness Agitation Sexual dysfunction
Anti-psychotics	Chlorpromazine (Thorazine) Haloperidol (Haldol) Risperidone (Risperdal) Olanzapine (Zyprexa) Quetiapine (Seroquel) Ziprasidone (Geodon) Aripiprazole (Abilify)	Bipolar disorder Schizophrenia Tourette's yndrome	Rigidity (muscular tension), Tremor, Tardive Dyskinesia (uncontrollable movements) Diabetes High cholesterol Weight gain Neuroleptic malignant syndrome (a life-threatening neurological disorder most often caused by an adverse reaction to antipsychotic drugs)
Hypnotics	Quazepam (Doral) Zolpidem (Ambien) Eszopiclone (Lunesta)	Insomnia Anxiety	Dependence Sleep walking
Mood stabilizers	Lithium Divalproex sodium (Depakote) Carbamazepine (Tegretol) Lamotrigine (Lamictal) Oxcarbazepine (Trileptal)	Bipolar disorder	Suicidal thoughts Loss of coordination Hallucinations Kidney, thyroid, liver, and pancreas damage Polycystic ovarian syndrome Weight gain

Source: NIMH, NIH, and our experts.

Note: The drug class categorizations and the corresponding examples of medications used in this analysis are intended to capture the common uses of psychotropic drugs and were reviewed by our experts. However, some of the drugs may have been developed and used for different purposes. For example, certain anti-anxiety drugs, such as benzodiazepines, may also be prescribed for insomnia. Similarly, some medications developed to treat depression, such as selective serotonin reuptake inhibitors (SSRIs) and tricyclic antidepressants, may also be used to treat anxiety disorders.

Higher Rates of Psychotropic Drug Prescriptions among Foster Children

Foster children in Florida, Massachusetts, Michigan, Oregon, and Texas were prescribed psychotropic drugs at rates 2.7 to 4.5 times higher than were nonfoster children in Medicaid in 2008.[14] The rates were higher among foster children for each of the age ranges—0 to 5 years old, 6 to 12 years old, and 13 to 17 years old—that we reviewed. See figure 1 for rates by state. Although a higher proportion of foster children received psychotropic drug prescriptions compared with nonfoster children, the vast majority of children receiving psychotropic drug prescriptions in these states were nonfoster children because the population of nonfoster children is much larger. In addition, according to our experts the higher rates of psychotropic drug prescriptions among foster children do not necessarily mean that the prescriptions were inappropriate; determining so would require, at minimum, a full review of each child's medical history.[15] Figure 1 shows prescription rates for children in each state for various age ranges. See appendix V for more information on psychotropic prescriptions to foster and nonfoster children in Medicaid.

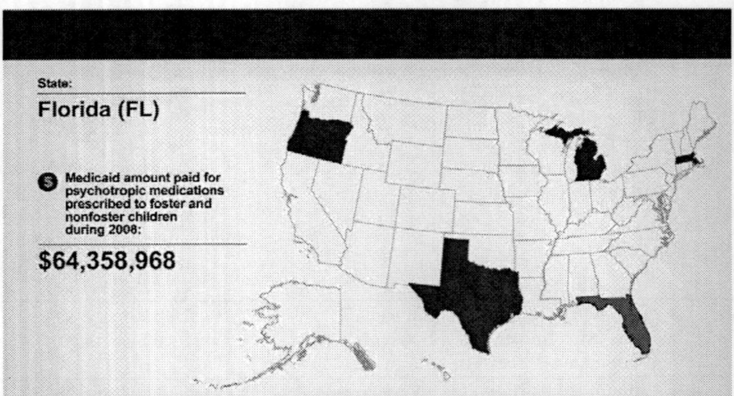

Percentage of children prescribed psychotropic medication age:	Foster children	Nonfoster children	Ratio of foster to nonfoster children
0–17 years old	22.0%	8.2%	2.7
13–17 years old	36.8%	11.9%	3.1
6–12 years old	31.2%	12.3%	2.5
0–5 years old	5.3%	3.3%	1.6

Note: Rates for foster and nonfoster children are comparable within the same state and the ratio of prescriptions to foster children to prescriptions to nonfoster children is comparable across states. However, prescription rates are not comparable across states because certain states covered more psychotropic drugs than other states. In addition, we excluded children whose prescriptions were not reported to CMS because they were covered by an HMO in the two states with both fee-for-service and HMO prescription coverage. Percentages and ratios are rounded to the nearest tenth, and therefore the reported ratio may be slightly different thanthe ratio of the rounded percentages.

Source: GAO analysis of state Medicaid and foster care data.

Figure 1. (Continued)

State:

Massachusetts (MA)

Medicaid amount paid for psychotropic medications prescribed to foster and nonfoster children during 2008:

$29,584,901

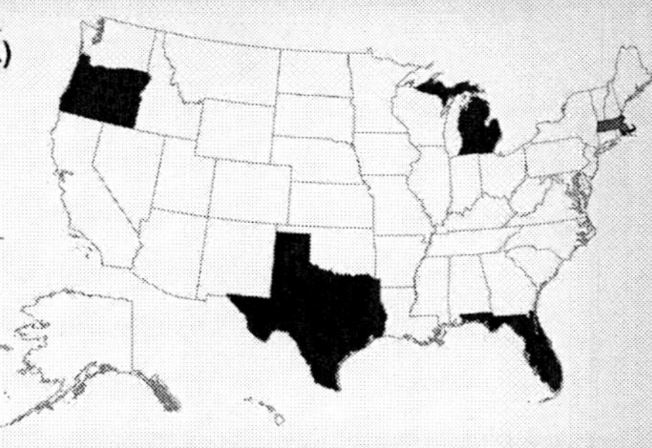

Percentage of children prescribed psychotropic medication age:	Foster children	Nonfoster children	Ratio of foster to nonfoster children
0–17 years old	39.1%	10.2%	3.8
13–17 years old	53.4%	14.7%	3.6
6–12 years old	44.8%	12.1%	3.7
0–5 years old	4.9%	2.2%	2.2

Note: Rates for foster and nonfoster children are comparable within the same state and the ratio of prescriptions to foster children to prescriptions to nonfoster children is comparable across states. However, prescription rates are not comparable across states because certain states covered more psychotropic drugs than other states. In addition, we excluded children whose prescriptions were not reported to CMS because they were covered by an HMO in the two states with both fee-for-service and HMO prescription coverage. Percentages and ratios are rounded to the nearest tenth, and therefore the reported ratio may be slightly different thanthe ratio of the rounded percentages.

Source: GAO analysis of state Medicaid and foster care data.

State:

Michigan (MI)

Medicaid amount paid for psychotropic medications prescribed to foster and nonfoster children during 2008:

$72,749,858

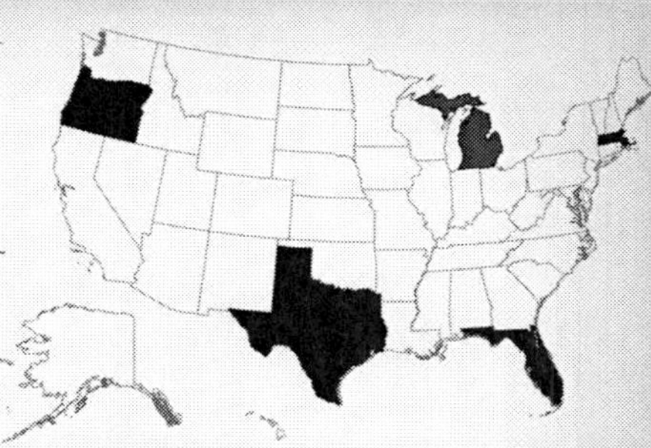

Percentage of children prescribed psychotropic medication age:	Foster children	Nonfoster children	Ratio of foster to nonfoster children
0–17 years old	21.0%	7.9%	2.7
13–17 years old	35.0%	13.1%	2.7
6–12 years old	26.7%	11.5%	2.3
0–5 years old	4.4%	1.1%	3.8

Note: Rates for foster and nonfoster children are comparable within the same state and the ratio of prescriptions to foster children to prescriptions to nonfoster children is comparable across states. However, prescription rates are not comparable across states because certain states covered more psychotropic drugs than other states. In addition, we excluded children whose prescriptions were not reported to CMS because they were covered by an HMO in the two states with both fee-for-service and HMO prescription coverage. Percentages and ratios are rounded to the nearest tenth, and therefore the reported ratio may be slightly different than the ratio of the rounded percentages.

Source. GAO analysis of state Medicaid and foster care data.

Figure 1. (Continued)

State:

Oregon (OR)

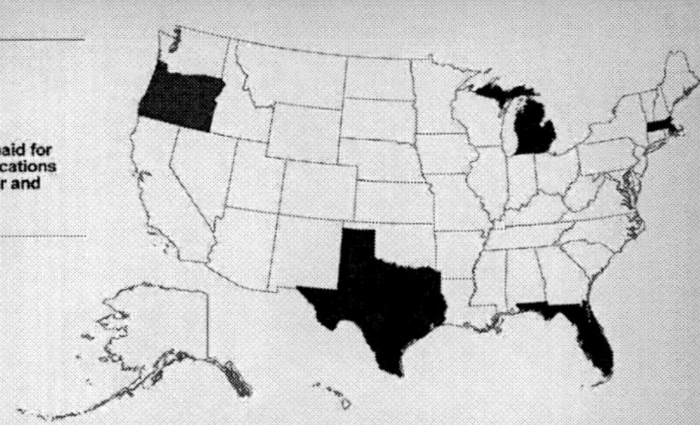

Medicaid amount paid for psychotropic medications prescribed to foster and nonfoster children during 2008:

$14,326,756

Percentage of children prescribed psychotropic medication age:	Foster children	Nonfoster children	Ratio of foster to nonfoster children
0–17 years old	19.7%	4.8%	4.1
13–17 years old	43.3%	12.0%	3.6
6–12 years old	23.4%	6.2%	3.8
0–5 years old	2.5%	0.6%	3.9

Note: Rates for foster and nonfoster children are comparable within the same state and the ratio of prescriptions to foster children to prescriptions to nonfoster children is comparable across states. However, prescription rates are not comparable across states because certain states covered more psychotropic drugs than other states. In addition, we excluded children whose prescriptions were not reported to CMS because they were covered by an HMO in the two states with both fee-for-service and HMO prescription coverage. Percentages and ratios are rounded to the nearest tenth, and therefore the reported ratio may be slightly different than the ratio of the rounded percentages.

Source: GAO analysis of state Medicaid and foster care data.

State:

Texas (TX)

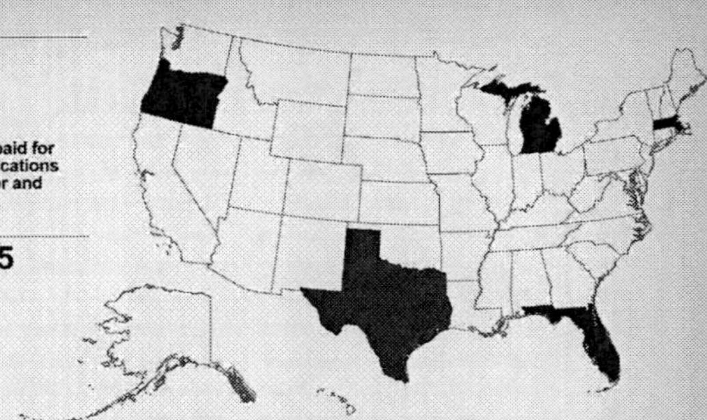

Medicaid amount paid for psychotropic medications prescribed to foster and nonfoster children during 2008:

$194,952,105

Percentage of children prescribed psychotropic medication age:	Foster children	Nonfoster children	Ratio of foster to nonfoster children
0–17 years old	32.2%	7.1%	4.5
13–17 years old	58.2%	11.4%	5.1
6–12 years old	45.8%	10.6%	4.3
0–5 years old	9.1%	3.1%	2.9

Note: Rates for foster and nonfoster children are comparable within the same state and the ratio of prescriptions to foster children to prescriptions to nonfoster children is comparable across states. However, prescription rates are not comparable across states because certain states covered more psychotropic drugs than other states. In addition, we excluded children whose prescriptions were not reported to CMS because they were covered by an HMO in the two states with both fee-for-service and HMO prescription coverage. Percentages and ratios are rounded to the nearest tenth, and therefore the reported ratio may be slightly different than the ratio of the rounded percentages.

Source: GAO analysis of state Medicaid and foster care data.

Figure 1. Psychotropic Prescription Rates for Children in Five States.

Through our interviews with state and federal officials and our experts, and our review of academic studies, we identified several factors that may contribute to these higher rates of prescribed psychotropic drug regimens. These factors included greater exposure to trauma before entering state care, frequent changes in foster placements, and varying state oversight policies. However, our literature search identified a relatively small number of studies that have been conducted to determine to what extent each of these factors contributes to higher prescription rates, or whether additional factors are involved.

Greater exposure to trauma. Research and interviews with certain state officials suggest that children entering foster care have more emotional and behavioral issues than do nonfoster children. For example, an analysis of 1996 service claims in one county revealed that 57 percent of foster children were diagnosed with a mental disorder—nearly 15 times that of nonfoster children receiving Medicaid assistance. ADHD, depression, and developmental disorders were the most common diagnoses.[16] According to the National Survey of Child and Adolescent Well-Being (NSCAW), 46 percent of children investigated by child welfare services (CWS) primarily came to the attention of CWS from a report of neglect, while 27 percent had experienced physical abuse as the most serious form of recorded maltreatment.[17] According to another study based on NSCAW data, approximately half of youths aged 2 to 14 years with completed child welfare investigations had clinically significant emotional or behavioral problems.[18]

State officials and our contracted child psychiatrists stated that higher levels of psychotropic drug prescriptions may be appropriate to deal with the increased prevalence and greater severity of mental health conditions among foster children. Further, Dr. Naylor noted that past trauma creates unique treatment challenges for those with multiple severe symptoms. In some cases, their symptoms do not clearly fit into existing diagnoses, which may cause them to receive multiple diagnoses that change with time, foster care placement, and medical provider. Dr. Naylor also noted that very little research has been done on the use of psychotropic drugs in foster children with severe symptoms. This limits the information available to providers on how best to treat their conditions. [19]

Frequent changes in foster placements. Foster children who change placements often do not have a consistent caretaker to plan treatment, offer consent, and provide oversight. As we have previously reported, changes in placement pose significant challenges for agencies, foster parents, and providers with regard to providing continuity of health care services and maintaining uninterrupted information on children's medical needs and courses of treatment.[20] Several studies of the use of psychotropic drugs have also noted that multiple foster care placements over short periods prevent an individual familiar with the child from coordinating and overseeing his or her long-term medical care.[21] Children entering foster care may lack medical care prior to entry, while children with prior medical care may have experienced disruptions in care and have missing or incomplete records. (We discuss how each of the six states oversees psychotropic drug prescriptions in the next section that discusses federal and state oversight of psychotropic drugs prescribed to foster children.)

Varying state oversight policies. States surveyed by the Tufts Clinical and Translational Science Institute in 2010 reported on several challenges that may affect prescribing patterns for foster children. These included a lack of collaboration among state agencies, professionals, and organizations responsible for the care of foster children; the consent process for foster children, which may require the input of multiple individuals or organizations; and the need for access to up-to-date guidelines on clinical practices regarding psychotropic prescriptions for foster children across stakeholder groups, including caregivers, child welfare agencies, schools, and prescribers. For example, the study found that 34 of 48 states had not implemented a system to identify prescriptions with dosages exceeding current maximum recommendations set by the product manufacturer, professional or federal standards, or state expert panels.[22]

Higher Rates of Potential Health Risk Indicators among Foster Children

In each of the five states analyzed, psychotropic prescription claims data for foster children showed higher rates of potential health risk indicators than those of nonfoster children in Medicaid. According to our experts, the following three prescribing practices carry increased levels of risk for children; concomitant prescriptions of five or more medications,[23] doses exceeding maximum levels in FDA-approved drug labels, and prescriptions for infants.[24] Figure 2 provides more information on these indicators by state.

State:

Florida (FL)

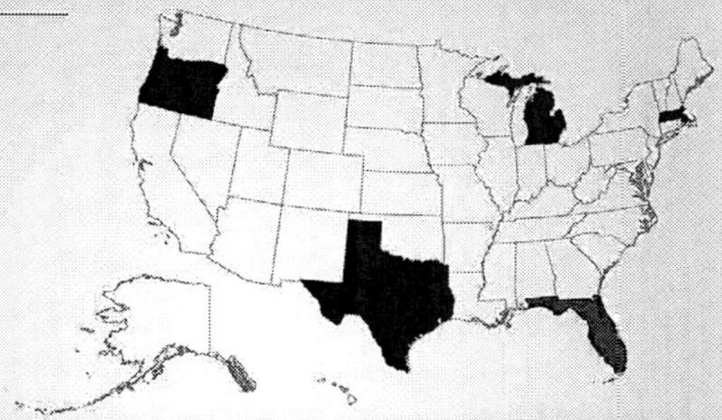

	Percentage of foster children	Percentage of nonfoster children
Children age 0–17 prescribed five (5) or more medications concomitantly	0.11%	0.03%
Children 0–17 with a dosage exceeding maximum guidelines based on FDA-approved labels	1.50%	0.44%
Children under 1 year old prescribed a psychotropic drug	2.1%	1.2%

Note: Rates for foster and nonfoster children are comparable within the same state and the ratio of prescriptions to foster children to prescriptions to nonfoster children is comparable across states. However, prescription rates are not comparable across states because certain states covered more psychotropic drugs than other states. In addition, we excluded children whose prescriptions were not reported to CMS because they were covered by an HMO in the two states with both fee-for-service and HMO prescription coverage.

Source: GAO analysis of state Medicaid and foster care data.

State:

Massachusetts (MA)

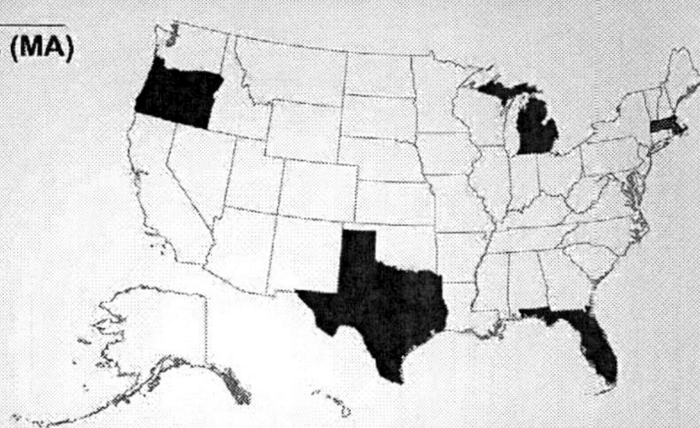

	Percentage of foster children	Percentage of nonfoster children
Children age 0–17 prescribed five (5) or more medications concomitantly	1.33%	0.07%
Children 0–17 with a dosage exceeding maximum guidelines based on FDA-approved labels	2.21%	0.56%
Children under 1 year old prescribed a psychotropic drug	0.7%	0.7%

Note: Rates for foster and nonfoster children are comparable within the same state and the ratio of prescriptions to foster children to prescriptions to nonfoster children is comparable across states. However, prescription rates are not comparable across states because certain states covered more psychotropic drugs than other states. In addition, we excluded children whose prescriptions were not reported to CMS because they were covered by an HMO in the two states with both fee-for-service and HMO prescription coverage.

Source: GAO analysis of state Medicaid and foster care data.

Figure 2. (Continued)

State:

Michigan (MI)

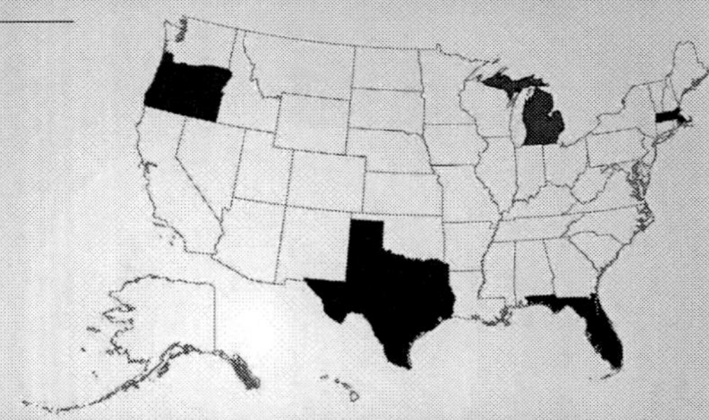

	Percentage of foster children	Percentage of nonfoster children
Children age 0–17 prescribed five (5) or more medications concomitantly	0.29%	0.02%
Children 0–17 with a dosage exceeding maximum guidelines based on FDA-approved labels	1.67%	0.49%
Children under 1 year old prescribed a psychotropic drug	1.5%	0.3%

Note: Rates for foster and nonfoster children are comparable within the same state and the ratio of prescriptions to foster children to prescriptions to nonfoster children is comparable across states. However, prescription rates are not comparable across states because certain states covered more psychotropic drugs than other states. In addition, we excluded children whose prescriptions were not reported to CMS because they were covered by an HMO in the two states with both fee-for-service and HMO prescription coverage.

Source: GAO analysis of state Medicaid and foster care data.

State:

Oregon (OR)

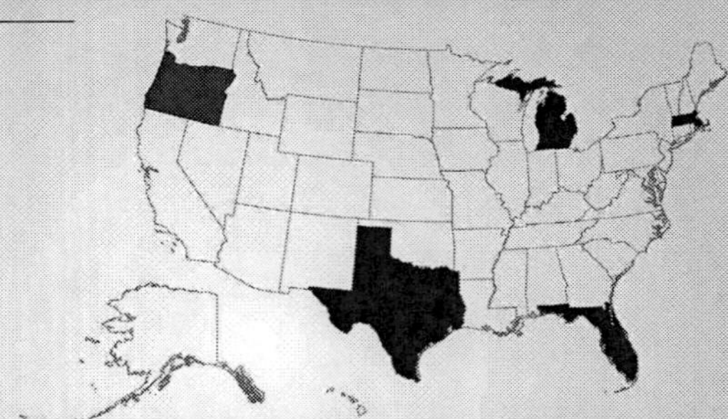

	Percentage of foster children	Percentage of nonfoster children
Children age 0–17 prescribed five (5) or more medications concomitantly	0.13%	0.01%
Children 0–17 with a dosage exceeding maximum guidelines based on FDA-approved labels	1.12%	0.16%
Children under 1 year old prescribed a psychotropic drug	0.3%	0.1%

Note: Rates for foster and nonfoster children are comparable within the same state and the ratio of prescriptions to foster children to prescriptions to nonfoster children is comparable across states. However, prescription rates are not comparable across states because certain states covered more psychotropic drugs than other states. In addition, we excluded children whose prescriptions were not reported to CMS because they were covered by an HMO in the two states with both fee-for-service and HMO prescription coverage.

Source: GAO analysis of state Medicaid and foster care data.

Figure 2. (Continued)

State:

Texas (TX)

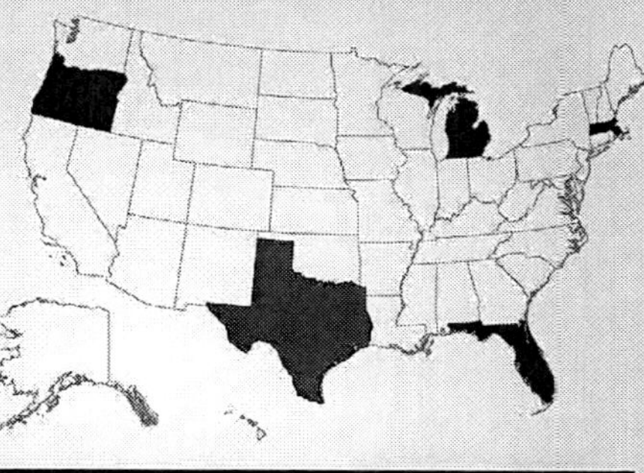

	Percentage of foster children	Percentage of nonfoster children
Children age 0–17 prescribed five (5) or more medications concomitantly	1.05%	0.02%
Children 0–17 with a dosage exceeding maximum guidelines based on FDA-approved labels	3.27%	0.37%
Children under 1 year old prescribed a psychotropic drug	1.2%	1.0%

Note: Rates for foster and nonfoster children are comparable within the same state and the ratio of prescriptions to foster children to prescriptions to nonfoster children is comparable across states. However, prescription rates are not comparable across states because certain states covered more psychotropic drugs than other states. In addition, we excluded children whose prescriptions were not reported to CMS because they were covered by an HMO in the two states with both fee-for-service and HMO prescription coverage.

Source: GAO analysis of state Medicaid and foster care data.

Figure 2. Psychotropic Drug Potential Health Risk Indicators for Five Selected States.

Concomitant psychotropic drug prescriptions.[25] Across the five states, the rate of children prescribed five or more psychotropic drugs concomitantly ranged from 0.11 to 1.33 percent among foster children compared with a lower 0.01 to 0.07 percent rate among nonfoster children. This translates to 1,752 children with such prescriptions in the five states—609 foster children and 1,143 nonfoster children. According to our experts, the use of five or more drugs at once is a high-risk practice. Our experts also said that no evidence supports the use of five or more psychotropic drugs in adults or children, and only limited evidence supports the use of even two drugs concomitantly in children. Increasing the number of drugs used concurrently increases the likelihood of adverse reactions and long-term side effects, such as high cholesterol or diabetes, and limits the ability to assess which of multiple drugs are related to a particular treatment goal.[26] See appendix VI for more information on concomitant prescription rates.

Doses Exceeding Maximum Levels in FDA-Approved Drug Labels. The rate of children prescribed medications exceeding maximum doses for the child's age as cited in the Texas Utilization Parameters, based on information in FDA-approved drug labels for the child's age ranged from 1.12 to 3.27 percent among foster children compared with a lower 0.16 to 0.56 percent rate among nonfoster children. 27 A total of 20,965 children in the five states had such a prescription—2,165 foster children and 18,800 nonfoster children. Of children prescribed drugs for which there was no FDA-recommended dose for their age, 0.34 to 1.52 percent of foster children and 0.05 to 0.16 percent of nonfoster children were prescribed dosages that exceeded the maximum standards published in the medical literature. According to our experts, taking drugs at dosages exceeding levels recommended by the FDA and medical literature increases the potential for adverse side effects. Although there may be cases in which such doses are clinically justified, in general, there is a lack of research demonstrating that high dosages are more effective. In addition, our experts said that for some drugs, a higher dose may be less effective than the more moderate recommended dose.[28] See appendix VII for information on rates of prescriptions above maximum doses for the child's age as cited in the Texas Utilization Parameters.

Table 2. Children Age 0-1 Year Old Prescribed Psychotropic Drugs in Five Selected States

Drug category (subclass)	Foster children	Nonfoster children
Anti-anxiety (antihistamines)[a]	55	3,454
Anti-anxiety (benzodiazepines)	17	254
Other anti-anxiety drugs	0	<10
ADHD drugs	<10	37
Antidepressants	<10	44
Antipsychotics	<10	12
Hypnotic	0	<10
Mood stabilizer	0	<10

Source: GAO analysis of state Medicaid and foster care data.

Note: A total of 76 foster children and 3,765 nonfoster children, or 3,841 children age 0 to 1, were prescribed a psychotropic drug. The totals in the table above do not add up to 3,841 because some infants were prescribed more than one psychotropic drug.

[a] Of children prescribed antihistamines, 26 foster children and 2,169 nonfoster children had prescriptions covering fewer than 20 days. According to one of our experts, this more likely represents a nonmental health use, such as for allergies or rashes.

Psychotropic prescriptions for infants. The rate of children under 1 year old prescribed a psychotropic drug ranged from 0.3 to 2.1 percent among foster children compared with a lower 0.1 to 1.2 percent rate among nonfoster children. This translates to 76 foster children and 3,765 nonfoster children under 1 year old in the five states—a total of 5,265 prescriptions.[29] Our experts said that there are no established mental health indications for the use of psychotropic drugs in infants, and providing them these drugs could result in serious adverse effects. According to our data, fewer than 10 infants in foster care and 22 nonfoster infants were prescribed clonidine—with dosages generally used in older children—which one of our experts said could result in significant sedation and potential cardiac problems including, on rare occasions, sudden death. Fewer than 10 infants in foster care were prescribed an antidepressant or an antipsychotic, compared with 44 and 12 infants not in foster care, respectively. According to our experts, antidepressants and antipsychotics have significant potential side effects, including cardiovascular and metabolic problems. Anti-anxiety drugs such as antihistamines and benzodiazepines accounted for the vast majority of the prescriptions for infants. Our experts noted that these drugs could have been prescribed for nonmental health conditions.[30] For example, the antihistamines could be prescribed to treat allergies, itching, and skin conditions such as eczema, the benzodiazepines for seizures or as sedation for a medical procedure. While physicians may use their discretion to prescribe these drugs to infants, these nonmental health uses still carry the same risk of adverse effects, including, for antihistamines, diminished mental alertness and excitation in young children. According to our experts, because infants are at a stage in their development where they are potentially more vulnerable to the effect of psychotropic drugs, these cases raise significant concerns and warrant further review. See table 2 and appendix VIII for more information.

Claims data also raise concerns about patient adherence to prescribed drug regimens, which our experts noted as a patient safety matter. Although foster children as a group were 1.7 to 3.3 times more likely to have three or more gaps of 7 to 29 days between prescriptions than nonfoster children, this is likely related to their overall higher rates of psychotropic prescriptions. When comparing only those prescribed psychotropic drugs, nonfoster children were 1.2 to 2.0 times more likely to have three or more gaps than foster children, suggesting that adherence is higher among foster children. Frequent gaps of 7 or more days in prescription claims have a number of potential causes, including a parent or caretaker's failure to fill prescriptions on behalf of a child in a timely manner or a lack of consistent access to care.[31] Gaps in drug claims do not indicate that the drugs as prescribed have potential health risks. However, nonadherence to drug regimens can pose significant risks to a patient, such as reduced efficacy from undertreatment, rebound of symptoms, and withdrawal symptoms. For example, the sudden discontinuation of benzodiazepines such as alprazolam can cause seizures[32] and the sudden discontinuation of SSRIs[33] such as paroxetine can cause a variety of problems, including dizziness, headaches, fatigue, and nausea.[34] Nonadherence to a drug regimen can cause the drug to appear ineffective even though it was not taken for a full trial. For example, antidepressants generally take 3 to 6 weeks to have a beneficial effect on the patient's symptoms.[35] Failure to take the antidepressant medications for a sufficient length of time may be interpreted as a lack of response to the treatment, which can result in the premature switch to or addition of other drugs. Table 3 and appendix IX provide more information on gaps in prescriptions for foster and nonfoster children by state.

Table 3. Percentage of Children Age 0-17 Prescribed a Psychotropic Drug with Three or More Gaps of 7-29 Days in Drug Claims in Five States

State	Percent of children who had three or more gaps in drug claims		Percent of children prescribed a psychotropic drug who had three or more gaps in drug claims	
	Foster children	Nonfoster children	Foster children	Nonfoster children
Florida	1.8	1.1	7.8	12.1
Massachusetts	3.4	1.8	8.4	16.4
Michigan	1.7	0.9	7.9	11.3
Oregon	1.6	0.5	7.7	9.5
Texas	2.2	0.7	6.6	8.6

Source: GAO analysis of Medicaid and foster care data for Florida, Massachusetts, Michigan, Oregon, and Texas.

[a] Since we used both primary and secondary lists in our gaps analysis, the number of foster and nonfoster children prescribed a psychotropic drug is slightly higher than reported in our overall prescription rates, which were based on primary drugs only.

Selected States' Psychotropic Drug Monitoring Programs Fall Short of AACAP-Best Principles Guidelines

Comparing the selected states' monitoring programs for psychotropic drugs provided to foster children with AACAP's guidelines indicates that, as of October 2011, each of the state programs falls short of providing comprehensive oversight as defined by AACAP. Though states are not required to follow these guidelines, the six states we examined developed monitoring programs that satisfied some of AACAP's best principles guidelines to varying degrees. Such variation is expected because states set their own oversight guidelines and have only recently been required, as a condition of receiving certain federal child welfare grants, to establish protocols for the appropriate use and monitoring of psychotropic drugs prescribed to foster children.[36]

HHS has provided limited guidance to the states on how to improve their control measures to monitor psychotropic drug prescriptions to foster children. Without formally endorsing specific oversight measures for states to implement, HHS conducts state reviews and provides other online resources, including the AACAP guidelines, to help states improve their programs. ACF performs child and family services reviews of states to ensure conformity with federal child welfare requirements—which include provisions for safety, permanency, and family and child wellbeing—and to assist states as they enhance their capacity to help families achieve positive outcomes.[37] These reviews included the examination of a limited number of children's case files, in part to determine whether the state foster care agency conducted assessments of children's mental health needs and provided appropriate services to address those needs. However, these reviews are not designed to identify specific potential health risk indicators related to psychotropic medications, and since they occur every 2 to 5 years, states cannot rely on these reviews to actively monitor prescriptions. In addition, ACF operates technical assistance centers and provides online resources such as links to state guidance on psychotropic drug oversight, academic studies on psychotropic drugs, and recordings of teleconferences related to the oversight of psychotropic drugs.[38] While HHS makes a variety of resources available to states developing oversight programs for psychotropic drugs, it has not endorsed any specific guidance. In the absence of HHS-endorsed guidance, states have developed varied oversight programs that in some cases fall short of AACAP's recommended guidelines.

The AACAP guidelines are arranged into four categories, including consent, oversight, consultation, and information sharing, that contain practices defined as minimal, recommended, or ideal. The following describes the extent to which the selected states' monitoring programs cover these areas. See appendix X for the full text of the AACAP guidelines and additional information on the selected states' practices consistent with these guidelines.

Consent: According to interviews and documentation provided by state Medicaid and foster care officials, all six selected states have implemented some practices consistent with AACAP guidelines for consent procedures, though in varying scope and application. According to AACAP, the consent process should be documented and monitored to ensure that caregivers are aware of relevant information, such as the child's diagnosis, expected benefits and risks of treatments, common side effects, and potentially severe adverse events. Thus, states that do not incorporate consent procedures similar to AACAP's guidelines may increase the likelihood that caregivers are not fully aware of the risks and benefits associated with the decision to medicate with psychotropic drugs, and may limit the caregiver's ability to accurately assess and monitor the foster child's reaction to the drugs. Table 4 lists AACAP's guidelines relative to consent and illustrates the extent to which states have implemented those guidelines.

Florida and Michigan provide examples of how states vary in their approach to monitoring consent procedures used for psychotropic drugs prescribed to foster children. For example, Florida requires all prescribers to obtain a standardized written consent form from the parental or legal guardian, or a court order, before a psychotropic drug is administered. The consent form includes the diagnosis, dosage, target symptoms, drug risks and benefits, drug monitoring plan, alternative treatment options, and discussions about the treatment between the child and the parent or legal guardian. Florida law identifies who is authorized to give consent, and obtains assent for psychotropic drug management from minors when age and developmentally appropriate. Florida provides required training to caseworkers, but the names and indications for use of commonly prescribed psychotropic drugs are not included.

In contrast, Michigan has policies identifying who is authorized to give consent to foster children, but does not use a standardized consent form that can be used to help inform consent decisions. Instead, Michigan requires that caseworkers maintain in their files the consent forms used by individual prescribers, which likely vary in content and may thus vary in helpfulness to consent-givers. Moreover, Michigan does not have training requirements in place to help caseworkers, court personnel, and foster parents become more effective advocates for children in their custody. Training for caseworkers is optional, but according to an agency official, the training was unavailable because no trainer had been hired as of September 2011. Michigan does not have policies for obtaining assent from minors when possible, thus meeting only one of AACAP's guidelines for consent procedures.

Oversight procedures: Each of the six states has developed some procedures similar to AACAP's guidelines for overseeing psychotropic drug prescriptions for foster children, as evidenced by interviews and documentation provided by state Medicaid and foster care officials.[39] According to one study, states that implement standards to improve oversight of the use of psychotropic drugs may create enhanced continuity of care, increased placement stability, reduced need for psychiatric hospitalization, and decreased incidence of adverse drug reactions.[40] As such, states that do not incorporate oversight procedures similar to AACAP's recommendations limit their ability to identify the extent to which potentially risky prescribing is occurring in the foster care population. Table 5 lists AACAP's guidelines relative to oversight and illustrates the extent to which selected states have implemented those guidelines.

Texas and Maryland provide examples of how states vary in their approach to oversight of psychotropic drug use among foster children. For example, the Texas Department of Family and Protective Services (DFPS) and the University of Texas at Austin College of Pharmacy assembled an advisory committee that included child and adolescent psychiatrists, psychologists, pediatricians, and other mental health professionals to develop psychotropic drug use parameters for foster children. These parameters are used to help identify cases requiring additional review. Factors that trigger additional reviews include dosages exceeding usual recommended levels, prescriptions for children of very young age, concomitant use of five or more psychotropic drugs, and prescriptions by a primary care provider lacking specialized training.41 According to the Texas foster care agency's data analysis, after Texas released these guidelines in 2005, psychotropic drug use among Texas foster care children declined from almost 30 percent in fiscal year 2004 to less than 21 percent in fiscal year 2010. Texas also analyzes Medicaid claims data to monitor psychotropic drug prescriptions for foster children and to identify any unusual prescribing behaviors. Texas provides quarterly reports to child welfare officials on the use of psychotropic drugs among foster children and treating clinicians have access to a child's medical records on a 24-hour basis.

Table 4. State Consent Laws and Policies Compared with AACAP's Best Principles Guidelines

Guideline		FL	MD	MA	MI	OR	TX
Minimal	Identify the parties empowered to consent for psychotropic drug treatment for youth in state custody in a timely fashion	Fully implemented	Fully implemented	Fully implemented	Fully implemented	Fully implemented	Fully implemented
Minimal	Establish a mechanism to obtain assent for psychotropic medication management from minors when possible	Fully implemented	Fully implemented	Not implemented	Not implemented	Not implemented	Fully implemented
Recommended	Obtain simply written psycho-educational materials and medication information sheets to facilitate the consent process	Fully implemented	Partially implemented	Fully implemented	Not implemented	Fully implemented	Fully implemented
Ideal	Establish training requirements for child welfare, court personnel and/or foster parents to help them become more effective advocates for children in their custody[a]	Partially implemented	Partially implemented	Partially implemented	Not implemented	Partially implemented	Fully implemented

Fully implemented
Partially implemented
Not implemented

FL Florida
MD Maryland
MA Massachusetts
MI Michigan
OR Oregon
TX Texas

Source: GAO analysis of information collected through interviews with, and various documentation provided by, the selected states' Medicaid and foster care officials, and the AACAP's best principles guideline.

[a]AACAP Best Principles Guidelines state this training should include the names and indications for use of commonly prescribed psychotropic medications, monitoring for medication effectiveness and side effects, and maintaining medication logs. Materials for this training should include a written "Guide to Psychotropic Medications" that includes many of the basic guidelines reviewed in the psychotropic medication training curriculum.

Table 5. State Oversight Laws and Policies Compared with AACAP's Best Principles Guidelines

Guideline		FL	MD	MA	MI	OR	TX
Minimal	Establish guidelines for the use of psychotropic medications for children in state custody	Partially implemented	Partially implemented	Partially implemented	Fully implemented	Not implemented	Fully implemented
Ideal	Oversight program includes an advisory committee to oversee a medication formulary and provide medication monitoring guidelines to practitioners who treat children in the child welfare system[a]	Partially implemented	Partially implemented	Not implemented	Partially implemented	Not implemented	Partially implemented
Ideal	Oversight program monitors the rate and types of psychotropic medication usage and the rate of adverse reactions among youth in state custody	Partially implemented	Partially implemented	Partially implemented	Partially implemented	Partially implemented	Partially implemented
Ideal	Oversight program establishes a process to review non-standard, unusual, and/or experimental psychiatric interventions with children who are in state custody	Partially implemented	Partially implemented	Partially implemented	Fully implemented	Partially implemented	Fully implemented
Ideal	Oversight program collects and analyzes data and makes quarterly reports to the state or county child welfare agency regarding the rates and types of psychotropic medication use. Make this data available to clinicians in the state to improve the quality of care provided	Partially implemented	Partially implemented	Partially implemented	Not implemented	Not implemented	Fully implemented
Ideal	Maintain an ongoing record of diagnoses, height and weight, allergies, medical history, ongoing medical problem list, psychotropic medications, and adverse medication reactions that are easily available to treating clinicians 24 hours a day	Partially implemented	Fully implemented	Partially implemented	Fully implemented	Partially implemented	Partially implemented

Fully implemented
Partially implemented
Not implemented

FL Florida
MD Maryland
MA Massachusetts
MI Michigan
OR Oregon
TX Texas

Source: GAO analysis of information collected through interviews with, and various documentation provided by, the selected states' Medicaid and foster care officials, and the AACAP's best principles guideline.

[a]AACAP describes advisory committees as composed of agency and community child and adolescent psychiatrists, pediatricians, other mental health providers, consulting clinical pharmacists, family advocates or parents, and state child advocates.

However, the electronic health record system does not always capture the child's height, weight, and allergies, which is optional for prescribers to enter into the system. This information is helpful as a child's weight may be used to determine the recommended dose for some medications, while allergy information may be used to determine whether a child should take a particular medication. In addition, ongoing medical problems are not recorded in the electronic health record system and Texas does not measure the rate of adverse reactions at the macro level among youth in state custody.

Maryland fully applies only one of the six AACAP guidelines for oversight procedures and partially applies others. Maryland provides foster children in out-of-home placement with a "medical passport" that serves as a record of the child's previous and current medical file. Each topic included in AACAP's guidelines for maintaining ongoing medical records, including diagnoses, allergies, and medical history, is documented in the passport, and an additional copy of the passport is kept in the child's case record and maintained electronically. However, Maryland has not produced any specific guidelines for the use of all psychotropic prescriptions among foster children, thus limiting the state's ability to identify potentially risky prescribing practices for the foster child population.[42] Without guidelines for psychotropic drugs, there are no criteria to help agency officials monitor the appropriateness of prescriptions. Moreover, Maryland does not review Medicaid claims data statewide specifically for foster children, and therefore does not produce quarterly reports to identify the rate and types of drugs used in the foster care population that could help identify and monitor prescribing trends. In addition, as stated earlier, Maryland's 2008 foster care data were found unreliable. Maryland officials told us that transitioning to a new records system in 2007 resulted in incorrect and missing data for foster children.

Consultation program: According to interviews and documentation provided by state Medicaid and foster care officials, five of the six states have implemented some of AACAP's guidelines for consultation, but only one of the six selected states has implemented a consultation program that ensures all consent-givers and prescribers are able to seek advice from child and adolescent psychiatrists before making consent decisions for foster children. States that do not have a consultation program to help link consent-givers and prescribers with child and adolescent psychiatrists may reduce the extent to which prescribers and consent-givers are informed about the expected benefits and risks of treatments, alternative treatments, and the risks associated with no treatment. Table 6 lists the AACAP guidelines relative to consultation programs and illustrates the extent to which selected states have implemented those guidelines.

Massachusetts and Oregon provide examples of how states vary their approach in providing expert consultations to caregivers. For example, Massachusetts' foster care agency started an initiative to connect child welfare staff to Medicaid pharmacists who can provide information on medications and the foster child's drug history, including interactions between any current and proposed drugs. In addition, primary care physicians who treat children, including foster care children, also have access to the state-funded Massachusetts Child Psychiatry Access Project, a system of regional children's mental health consultation teams designed to help pediatricians find and consult with child psychiatrists. Massachusetts has six child psychiatrists who are available to provide consultations on a part-time basis to child welfare staff, but these consultations are not available for other consent-givers such as foster parents. The foster care agency's consultation program also provides face-to-face evaluations of foster children at the request of consent-givers concerned about a child's treatment.

Table 6. State Consultation Programs Compared with AACAP's Best Principles Guidelines

Guideline		FL	MD	MA	MI	OR	TX
Recommended	Design a consultation program administered by child and adolescent psychiatrists. This program provides consultation by child and adolescent psychiatrists to the persons or agency that is responsible for consenting for treatment with psychotropic medications	Fully implemented	Not implemented	Partially implemented	Not implemented	Partially implemented	Partially implemented
Recommended	The consultation program provides consultations by child and adolescent psychiatrists to, and at the request of, physicians treating this difficult patient population	Fully implemented	Partially implemented	Fully implemented	Not implemented	Not implemented	Not implemented
Recommended	The consultation program conducts face-to-face evaluations of youth by child and adolescent psychiatrists at the request of the child welfare agency, the juvenile court, or other state or county agencies empowered by law to consent for treatment with psychotropic medications when concerns have been raised about the pharmacological regimen	Not implemented	Not implemented	Fully implemented	Not implemented	Not implemented	Fully implemented

Fully implemented
Partially implemented
Not implemented

FL Florida
MD Maryland
MA Massachusetts
MI Michigan
OR Oregon
TX Texas

Source: GAO analysis of information collected through interviews with, and various documentation provided by, the selected states' Medicaid and Foster Care officials, and the AACAP's best principles guideline.

In early 2009, Oregon put a consultation program in place to help consent-givers make informed decisions. In 2010, Oregon's foster care agency shifted the responsibility for all consent decisions where the agency has legal custody or is the legal guardian of the child from foster parents to child welfare agency officials, who now have access to a child and adolescent psychiatrist and can seek consultations before making consent decisions. However, the consultation program does not conduct face-to-face evaluations of children—by a child and adolescent psychiatrist—at the request of consent-givers, nor does it enable prescribing physicians to consult with child and adolescent psychiatrists. Oregon has plans for the development of the Oregon Psychiatric Access Line for Kids, which would allow primary care physicians and nurse practitioners to consult with child psychiatrists, but agency officials told us the program is not operational due to a lack of funding.

Information sharing: Four of the six selected states have created websites with information on psychotropic drugs for clinicians, foster parents, and other caregivers. Access to comprehensive information could help ensure that clinicians, foster parents, and other interested parties are fully informed about the use and management of psychotropic drugs. Table 7 lists AACAP's guidelines relative to information sharing and illustrates the extent to which selected states have implemented those guidelines.

For example, Florida's foster care agency has partnered with the University of South Florida to implement Florida's Center for the Advance-ment of Child Welfare Practice to provide needed information and support to Florida's professional child welfare stakeholders.[43] The program's website is consistent with four of AACAP's six guidelines for information sharing. For example, the website includes policies and procedures governing psychotropic drug management, staff publications and educational materials about psychotropic drugs, consent forms, and links to other informative publications and news stories related to foster children and psychotropic drugs. However, the website does not provide reports on prescription patterns for psychotropic drugs or adverse effect rating forms.

In comparison, Oregon's foster care agency developed a website that includes information regarding psychotropic medication, but the website is not updated regularly to operate as an ongoing information resource. The website currently has information on state policies and procedures governing the use of psychotropic drugs and also contains web links to consent forms and a medication chart that can be used as a psychotropic medication reference tool. However, the website does not meet three of the six information-sharing guidelines, including those on posting adverse effect rating forms, reporting prescription patterns, and providing links to other informative websites. States with less accessibility to comprehensive information may limit the extent to which physicians, foster parents, and other interested parties are informed about the use and management of psychotropic drugs.

Table 7. State Information-sharing Laws and Policies Compared with AACAP's Best Principles Guidelines

Guideline		FL	MD	MA	MI	OR	TX
Ideal	Create a website to provide ready access for clinicians, foster parents, and other caregivers to pertinent policies and procedures governing psychotropic medication management	Fully implemented	Not implemented	Fully implemented	Not implemented	Fully implemented	Fully implemented
Ideal	Website includes psycho-educational materials	Fully implemented	Not implemented	Fully implemented	Not implemented	Fully implemented	Fully implemented
Ideal	Website includes consent forms	Fully implemented	Not implemented	Not implemented	Not implemented	Fully implemented	Not implemented
Ideal	Website includes adverse effect rating forms	Not implemented	Not implemented	Not implemented	Not implemented	Not implemented	Not implemented
Ideal	Website includes reports on prescription patterns for psychotropic medications	Not implemented	Not implemented	Not implemented	Not implemented	Not implemented	Fully implemented
Ideal	Website includes links to helpful, accurate, and ethical websites about child and adolescent psychiatric diagnoses and psychotropic medications	Fully implemented	Not implemented	Not implemented	Not implemented	Not implemented	Fully implemented

Fully implemented
Partially implemented
Not implemented

FL Florida
MD Maryland
MA Massachusetts
MI Michigan
OR Oregon
TX Texas

Source: GAO analysis of information collected through interviews with, and various documentation provided by, the selected states' Medicaid and Foster Care officials, and the AACAP's best principles guideline.

CONCLUSION

The higher rates of psychotropic drug prescriptions among foster children may be explained by their greater mental health needs and the challenges inherent to the foster care system. However, thousands of foster and nonfoster children in the five states we analyzed were found to have prescriptions that carry potential health risks. While doctors are permitted to prescribe these drugs under current laws, increasing the number of drugs used concurrently and exceeding the maximum recommended dosages for certain psychotropic drugs have been shown to increase the risk of adverse side effects in adults. Psychotropic prescriptions for infants are also of concern, due to the potential for serious adverse effects even when these drugs are used for nonmental health purposes. Comprehensive oversight programs would help states identify these and other potential health risks and provide caregivers and prescribers with the information necessary to weigh drug risks and benefits. The recently enacted Child and Family Services Improvement and Innovation Act requires states that apply for certain child welfare grants to establish protocols for monitoring psychotropic drugs prescribed to foster children. Under the act, each state is authorized to develop its own monitoring protocols, but HHS-endorsed, nationwide guidelines for consent, oversight, consultation, and information sharing could help states close the oversight gaps we identified and increase protections for this vulnerable population.

Recommendation for Executive Action

To improve the comprehensiveness of oversight of psychotropic drugs prescribed to foster children, we recommend that the Secretary of HHS evaluate our findings and consider endorsing guidance to state Medicaid and child welfare agencies on best practices for monitoring psychotropic drug prescriptions for foster children, including guidance that addresses, at minimum, informed consent, oversight, consultation, and information sharing.

Agency Comments and Our Evaluation

We provided a draft copy of this report to HHS and the state foster care and Medicaid agencies of the six selected states for their review. We also received e-mails with comments from officials from Florida Department of Children and Families (DCF), Maryland Department of Human Resources (DHR), and Michigan Department of Community Health (DCH), which we describe below. HHS and certain states also provided technical comments, which we incorporated as appropriate.

HHS agreed with our recommendation and stated that ACF will issue guidance to the states on best practices for monitoring psychotropic drug prescriptions for foster children. In addition, ACF will disseminate to states the current best practices for use in developing their approaches and protocols.

We strongly support these steps and encourage HHS to follow through on these actions. The comment letters from the states generally provided clarifications or further information on specific aspects of each state program, which we incorporated, as appropriate.

In an e-mail response from the Chief of Quality Assurance, the Florida DCF, which administers the state's foster care program, stated that our report appeared factually correct based on the data sources. Florida DCF stated that our statement that thousands of foster and nonfoster infants were prescribed psychotropic medications seemed inflammatory, given that the number of infants in foster care represented was less than 100 and the report is focused on foster children. Florida DCF also noted that the state has very few cases of foster children under 1 year old prescribed a psychotropic drug, and stated that they had confirmed that all but one had a documented medical reason for the prescription. We continue to believe that the inclusion of both foster and non-foster children in our total is appropriate, given the serious adverse effects these drugs may have in infants. We did not review case records for these children as part of this review, and thus cannot conclude whether there is a medical justification for these prescriptions.

In an e-mail response from the deputy executive director of operations of the Maryland DHR, the agency stated that it regretted that its foster care data had not been usable for this report. Maryland DHR stated that it engaged in data cleanup and improvement following the 2007 launch of its new information system. The agency also stated that it would be helpful to Maryland, and perhaps other states, to make use of our methodology and tools for further analysis. Maryland DHR would like to make use of our analysis tools for its 2010 or 2011 foster care data, which Maryland stated have much higher accuracy than the data available in 2008. The agency agreed with the need to have comprehensive oversight programs and established protocols for monitoring psychotropic drugs prescribed to foster children, but the costs of implementing oversight mechanisms must be supported in order for these new guidelines to be effective. We would be willing to share our methodology with Maryland and any other state to help them improve the monitoring of children using psychotropic medications. We also agree that additional oversight mechanisms may require additional resources to be effective.

In an e-mail response from the director of the office of audit, Michigan DCH agreed with the recommendation and anticipated additional federal resources to be able to comply with future requirements.

Gregory D. Kutz
Director
Forensic Audits and Investigative Service

List of Requesters
The Honorable Thomas R. Carper
Chairman
Subcommittee on Federal Financial Management,
Government Information, Federal Services, and International Security
Committee on Homeland Security and Governmental Affairs
United States Senate

The Honorable Susan M. Collins
Ranking Member
Committee on Homeland Security and Governmental Affairs
United States Senate
The Honorable Scott P. Brown
Ranking Member
Subcommittee on Federal Financial Management, Government
Information, Federal Services, and International Security
Committee on Homeland Security and Governmental Affairs
United States Senate

The Honorable Charles E. Grassley Ranking Member
Committee on the Judiciary
United States Senate

The Honorable John McCain
United States Senate

APPENDIX I. OBJECTIVES, SCOPE, AND METHODOLOGY

Our objectives were to: (1) compare rates of psychotropic drug prescriptions in foster children and nonfoster children covered by Medicaid in 2008, including indicators of potential health risks, and (2) examine federal and state oversight policies in effect for psychotropic drugs prescribed to foster children through October 2011.

To determine the rate of psychotropic drug prescriptions to foster and nonfoster children enrolled in Medicaid, we obtained Medicaid Statistical Information System (MSIS) claims data for prescriptions adjudicated between January 1 and December 31, 2008, for six selected states— Florida, Maryland, Massachusetts, Michigan, Oregon, and Texas.[44] At the start of our audit, 2008 data were the most recent calendar year prescription claims data available from Centers for Medicare & Medicaid Services (CMS). We selected these states based on the following factors: (1) existence of a fee-for-service prescription or carve-out program reporting psychotropic drug prescription data to CMS,[45] (2) geographic diversity, and (3) state foster care program size. The audit was limited to data on children in a Medicaid fee-for-service prescription or carve-out program for psychotropic drugs and may not generalize to other states or populations.

We obtained data on persons enrolled in Medicaid and/or receiving Medicaid services during calendar year 2008, and children in foster care during calendar year 2008, from the respective agencies in each of the six selected states. We identified psychotropic prescription claims for foster children and nonfoster children by matching the MSIS claims data with the Medicaid and foster care files and using national drug code information in the Medicaid data. For the purpose of our analysis, we defined foster children as any child under age 18 as of July 1, 2008, and in foster care for a period of 30 or more consecutive days during calendar year 2008, and excluded children in foster care less than 30 days during 2008 from our analysis. We included only claims filled while the child was in foster care. We defined nonfoster children as any child under age 18 as of July 1, 2008, not in foster care at any time during calendar year 2008. Due to a small percentage of missing or incorrect identifiers in the foster care data, some children from the Medicaid files could not be correctly matched to foster care records. The result is an underestimate of the number of foster children and an overestimate of nonfoster children.

We developed a list of psychotropic drugs likely to be prescribed in the six selected states by reviewing each state's list of approved drugs, and a list of psychotropic drugs published by the National Institute of Mental Health (NIMH).[46] We verified the active ingredient for each drug in databases published by the Food and Drug Administration (FDA) or Thomson Reuters. The list was then reviewed by our two contracted child psychiatrists with clinical and research experience in the prescription of psychotropic drugs to children. Based on their recommendations, we developed a primary list of psychotropic drugs comprised of attention deficit hyperactivity disorder (ADHD) drugs, antidepressants, certain anti- anxiety drugs, antipsychotics, combination drugs, hypnotics, and mood stabilizers for our analysis of prescription rates of at least one psychotropic medication, and dosages exceeding FDA maximum recommended therapeutic doses. We counted a prescription for any primary drug in our analysis of prescription rates; we did not require that the prescription cover a minimum number of days.[47] We also developed a secondary list of drugs—anticonvulsants, antiparkinson drugs, antienuretics, sleep aids, and certain anti-anxiety drugs—for our analysis of concomitant prescriptions. When paired with a primary psychotropic drug, these medications counted toward the total number of drugs prescribed concomitantly. When used alone or in combination with other secondary medications, they did not count as concomitant prescriptions.[48] This may result in a slight underestimate of the prescription of concomitant psychotropic drugs; however, this should not differ between the foster and nonfoster care populations. These MSIS prescription claims data do not include diagnosis codes, and therefore, we cannot be sure that all the drugs in our analysis were prescribed for mental health purposes. By eliminating secondary drugs such as anticonvulsants from our analysis of prescription rates for one or more drugs, we likely understate the percentage of children prescribed psychotropic drugs for mental health purposes. We used both our primary and secondary lists when examining gaps in medications.

The five states differed in the types of prescriptions included in the claims data we analyzed. Because Medicaid is a state-administered program, each state has its own formulary of the drugs that it covers, including which drugs are covered by its fee for service or through its managed care. Generally, prescription claims paid for on a fee-for-service basis were reported to CMS by the five states during 2008, and therefore were included in the data we obtained from CMS and analyzed. In Florida and Massachusetts, prescriptions for those individuals not enrolled in a health maintenance organization (HMO) were reported to CMS, and we analyzed only these children.[49] In addition, we found certain states through their formularies and prescription drug carve outs covered more drugs from our psychotropic list than other states. As such, while rates of psychotropic prescriptions are not comparable across states, they are comparable between foster and nonfoster children within the same state. Similarly, the ratio of prescriptions to foster children to prescriptions to nonfoster children is comparable across states.

We used MSIS prescription claims data to calculate the total amount paid by state Medicaid programs for prescriptions on the primary list of psychotropic drugs used in our analysis for children in foster care for 30 days or more and nonfoster children in Medicaid during 2008. This amount paid includes only claims paid for by a fee-for-service program and does not include manufacturer rebates or other costs such as managed care. We obtained additional information about drug dosages and administration routes from Thomson Reuters' Red Book.[50] We did not evaluate relative rates of usage for brand name and generic drugs in our analysis.

We examined the concomitant prescription of five or more drugs with unique active ingredients. We did not allow for overlapping prescriptions of the same drug. We counted a drug as prescribed continuously if within 3 consecutive calendar months, the prescription(s) had at least 84 days supply within that time period. Requiring a minimum of 84 days resulted in a more conservative estimate of concomitant prescriptions by eliminating cases in which a patient was prescribed a new drug without finishing the previous supply, thereby creating the appearance of concurrent use. For example, when one or more prescriptions for the same drug were filled before the days' supply of the previous prescription had elapsed, we assumed that the subsequent prescriptions had been saved and used in sequence, with no overlapping days. Where the total days supply exceeded 84 days for a 3-month consecutive period, we counted this as continuous use.[51] We added the number of unique active ingredients prescribed continuously for each 3-month period (i.e., two kinds of the same drug counted as one active ingredient). We did not count concomitant prescriptions of a brand name and generic drug with the same active ingredient.

We developed indicators of potential health risks based on input from our child psychiatrists; a literature review; state guidelines; and interviews with officials from CMS, state Medicaid and foster care offices, NIMH, and professional medical associations. The final indicators of potential health risks were: concomitant prescriptions of five or more drugs, prescriptions exceeding dosage guidelines in the Psychotropic Medication Utilization Parameters for Texas Foster Children, and psychotropic prescriptions to children under 1 year old. In addition, we evaluated gaps of 7 to 29 days in prescriptions of a drug to identify non adherence to drug regimens, which can pose significant risks to a patient. Analysis of only 1 year of claims data prevented us from determining whether a single drug was tried before adding additional drugs in all cases. Additionally, data limitations prevented us from comparing prescribing patterns for foster youth in different settings, and lack of pharmacy claims for hospitalized youth prevented us from examining prescribing patterns for these children or comparing hospitalized foster and nonfoster youth.

To determine whether children were prescribed psychotropic drugs exceeding FDA maximum recommended therapeutic doses for their age or standards published in medical literature for their age, we used the dosage guidelines in the 2010 Texas Utilization Parameters. We excluded anti-convulsants and dosages based on the child's weight from our analysis. To identify children for whom there was no FDA-recommended dose and who exceeded the next relevant standard, we defined the next relevant standard as the published guidelines for the child's age or next highest age range, the FDA-recommended dose for the next highest age range, or the published standards for a different version of the drug (i.e., standards for the extended release version of the drug). We calculated rates of psychotropic prescriptions to children age 0 to 1 in the same way that we calculated psychotropic prescription rates for other age groups. See discussion above for definition of foster children and nonfoster children and the kinds of drugs included in this analysis.

We also examined drugs prescribed to foster or nonfoster children to identify gaps in the dispensing of the drugs. In consultation with our experts, we defined a gap in prescriptions as 7 to 29 days between the last day of the first prescription and the fill date of the next prescription. We examined gaps across prescriptions for the same active ingredient, regardless of dosage. Similar to our concomitant analysis, when one or more prescriptions for the same drug were filled before the days supply of the previous prescription had elapsed, we assumed that the subsequent prescriptions had been saved and used in sequence, with no overlapping days. This methodology may understate gaps for patients with two prescriptions for different versions of the same medication, such as a drug and its extended release version. In this case, a break in one of the medications would not appear as a gap if the prescription for the other drug continued to be filled. Conversely, prescribers may reduce the dosage of a medication without writing a new prescription, which could appear as a gap in prescriptions. For example, if a patient had been prescribed two 10 mg doses per day, and was adjusted down to a single dose of 10 mg per day, the next prescription would be filled later than expected, appearing as a gap. Finally, children who exited and reentered Medicaid in a 30-day period during the course of the year would appear to have a gap in their prescriptions. If a child had three such gaps, he or she would have been included in the rate of children with three or more gaps in a medication, although it is not possible to know from prescription claims data whether the child had other prescription coverage during the time he or she was not in Medicaid.

To identify federal requirements and guidance related to the oversight of psychotropic drugs, we interviewed officials from CMS and the Administration for Children and Families (ACF), and reviewed laws and regulations.

To determine the design of controls over psychotropic medications prescribed to foster children in each of the six selected states, we reviewed state statutes and policies or regulations related to the prescription of psychotropic drugs to foster children, and interviewed officials from the six selected states' Medicaid and child welfare agencies. Finally, we interviewed officials from the American Academy of Child and Adolescent Psychiatry (AACAP) to obtain an understanding of their methods for developing best practice guidelines for providing psychotropic drugs to foster children. We selected AACAP's "Position Statement on Oversight of Psychotropic Medication Use for Children in State Custody: A Best Principles Guideline" as a standard against which to compare state program frameworks based on a literature review and our discussions with officials from NIMH and CMS. However, states have legal discretion to administer Medicaid and foster care programs, and are not required to implement controls based on these best principles guidelines.

We performed this audit from February 2010 through November 2011 in accordance with generally accepted government auditing standards. Those standards require that we plan and perform the audit to obtain sufficient, appropriate evidence to provide a reasonable basis for our findings and conclusions based on our audit objectives. We believe that the evidence obtained provides a reasonable basis for our findings and conclusions based on our audit objectives.

We performed data checks to determine the reliability of the MSIS prescription claims data provided by CMS, state Medicaid files provided by Medicaid agencies in the six selected states, databases of children in foster care provided by child welfare agencies in the six selected states, and Thomson Reuters Red Book. While a small number of Medicaid and foster care records may contain inaccurate personal data or prescription information likely resulting from data entry errors, based on our discussions with agency officials and our own testing, we concluded that the data elements in five of the six states used for this report were sufficiently reliable to address our audit objectives. However, we determined through data tests, interviews, and reviews of state audit reports that data on children in Maryland foster care during 2008 were unreliable. For example, our electronic tests of Maryland data found 8,869 children in foster care as of September 30, 2008—16 percent more than the 7,613 children that Maryland reported to ACF for that year. In addition, state audits in 2008 reported duplicate records with different identifying numbers for the same child, records showing children who had exited foster care as still enrolled in the program, and personal information for the parent recorded as that of the child. We therefore concluded that the

Maryland foster care data were unreliable and excluded Maryland from our analysis of rates of psychotropic prescriptions.

APPENDIX II. USES AND SIDE EFFECTS OF PSYCHOTROPIC DRUGS[52]

Psychotropic drugs are used to treat the symptoms of mental health conditions such as schizophrenia, depression, bipolar disorder (sometimes called manic-depressive illness), anxiety disorders, and ADHD. These drugs cannot cure mental disorders, but they can treat the symptoms to help people feel better so they can function. For our analyses, we included drugs in the following categories: (1) ADHD, (2) anti-anxiety, (3) antidepressants, (4) anti-psychotics, (5) hypnotics, and (6) mood stabilizers and any medications that combine two or more of these categories.[53] The following information was taken primarily from NIMH's 2008 Mental Health Medications guide, and provides the common uses and potential side effects for each type of psychotropic drug:[54]

Attention Deficit Hyperactivity Disorder (ADHD) drugs are prescribed to individuals who are hyperactive, impulsive, and easily distracted. These drugs are used to help individuals focus, work, and learn, and may also improve physical coordination. These drugs include nonstimulant drugs such as atomoxetine (Strattera), guanfacine (Intuniv), and clonidine (Kapvay), and stimulant drugs such as methylphenidate (Ritalin, Metadate, Concerta, Daytrana), amphetamine (Adderall), and lisdexamfetamine dimesylate (Vyvanse). Stimulants can cause side effects such as decreased appetite and sleep problems, and less frequently, tics or personality changes. Most minor side effects can be eliminated by lowering the drug dosage. More seriously, there are possible rare side effects associated with the use of ADHD drugs. ADHD patients also have a slightly higher risk for drug-related psychiatric side effects, such as hearing voices, having hallucinations, becoming paranoid, or becoming manic.

Anti-anxiety drugs are prescribed to individuals to treat post-traumatic stress disorder, generalized anxiety disorder, obsessive compulsive disorder, panic disorder, and social phobias. Benzodiazepines, one type of anti-anxiety drug, include drugs such as clonazepam (Klonopin), lorazepam (Ativan), and alprazolam (Xanax).[55] The most common side effects for benzodiazepines are drowsiness and dizziness. Other side effects include upset stomach, blurred vision, headache, confusion, grogginess, and nightmares. Another anti-anxiety drug used to treat generalized anxiety disorders is buspirone (Buspar).[56] Unlike benzodiazepines, however, it takes at least 2 weeks for buspirone to begin working. Possible side effects of buspirone include dizziness, headaches, nausea, nervousness, lightheadedness, excitement, and trouble sleeping.

Antidepressants are prescribed to treat individuals who suffer from depression. All antidepressants contain an FDA box warning—the most serious type of warning—to alert users to the increased risk of suicidal thinking or attempts in children, adolescents, and young adults taking this type of drug.

Older antidepressant medications cause more side effects than newer classes of antidepressants, but they may be the best medication for some people. Older generations of antidepressants include tricyclics and tetracyclics, such as protriptyline (Vivactil) and trimipramine (Surmontil), and monoamine oxidase inhibitors (MAOIs), such as isocarboxazid (Marplan) and phenelzine (Nardil). These drugs can cause side effects such as dry mouth, constipation, bladder problems, sexual problems, blurred vision, and drowsiness. MAOIs can interact with various foods or drugs high in tyramine—including certain cheeses, wines, pickles, and over-the-counter medications—to produce severe hypertension.

Other types of antidepressants include selective serotonin reuptake inhibitors (SSRIs) such as fluoxetine (Prozac) and sertraline (Zoloft), and serotonin and norepinephrine reuptake inhibitors (SNRIs) such as venlafaxine (Effexor) and duloxetine (Cymbalta). SSRIs and SNRIs can cause side effects such as agitation, serotonin syndrome, and sexual dysfunction, as well as headache, nausea, and sleeplessness or drowsiness when the patient first begins taking the drugs. Another type of antidepressant that acts on the neurotransmitter dopamine is called bupropion (Wellbutrin). Bupropion can cause side effects such as drowsiness, dry mouth, dizziness, headache, nausea, seizures, chest pain, and confusion.

Antipsychotic drugs are used to treat schizophrenia, bipolar disorders, irritability in autism, and depression. The first generation of antipsychotics, also known as "typical" antipsychotics, includes chlorpromazine (Thorazine) and haloperidol (Haldol). Typical antipsychotics can cause side effects such as rigidity, persistent muscle spasms, tremors, and restlessness and, with long-term use, tardive dyskinesia. The second generation of antipsychotics, or "atypical" antipsychotics, includes risperidone (Risperdal), quetiapine (Sero quel), and aripiprazole (Abilify). While typical antipsychotics are more likely to cause movement disorders, such as uncontrollable muscle spasms that in some cases cannot be cured , atypical antipsychotics can cause weight gain and changes in metabolism, potentially leading to an increased risk of diabetes and high cholesterol. Both typical and atypical antipsychotics can also cause drowsiness, dizziness when changing positions, blurred vision, rapid heartbeat, sensitivity to the sun, skin rashes, and menstrual problems.

Hypnotics cause sleep or partial loss of consciousness, and are used to treat insomnia and some anxiety disorders. Benzodiazepine hypnotics include drugs such as flurazepam (Dalmane), quazepam (Doral), and triazolam (Halcion).[57] Benzodiazepine hypnotics can be addictive and are associated with side effects such as daytime drowsiness, a hungover feeling, and the worsening of certain breathing problems. Nonbenzodiazepine hypnotics include drugs such as Zaleplon (Sonata), Zolpidem (Ambien), and Eszopiclone (Lunesta). These hypnotics may be less addictive than benzodiazepines but can cause side effects such as driving, making phone calls, or eating while asleep.

Mood stabilizers are drugs used to treat individuals with bipolar disorder (also known as manic-depressive illness). Lithium and anticonvulsant drugs can both be used as mood stabilizers.

Lithium was the first mood stabilizer approved by the FDA in the 1970s for treating both manic and depressive episodes. Lithium can cause several side effects, and some of them may become serious. These side effects include: loss of coordination, excessive thirst, frequent urination, blackouts, seizures, slurred speech, irregular or pounding heartbeat, hallucinations, changes in vision, rashes, swelling of the face or limbs, and low thyroid function (hypothyroidism).

Anticonvulsant drugs are also used as mood stabilizers. These drugs were originally developed to treat seizures, but they were found to help control moods as well. One anticonvulsant commonly used as a mood stabilizer is divalproex sodium (Depakote). Other anticonvulsants used as mood stabilizers are carbamazepine (Tegretol), lamotrigine (Lamictal) and oxcarbazepine (Trileptal). Like antidepressants, these drugs also have an FDA warning to alert users to the increased risk of suicidal thinking or behaviors in individuals taking this type of drug. Some other serious side effects of these drugs include damage to the liver and pancreas (divalproex sodium), polycystic ovarian syndrome (divalproex sodium), and serious skin rash (lamotrigine).

APPENDIX III. LIST OF PSYCHOTROPIC DRUGS USED IN ANALYSIS

The following table lists the type of psychotropic drug and drug ingredients for all drugs used in the analysis.

Table 8. Psychotropic Drugs Used in Analysis

Type of psychotropic drug	Psychotropic drug ingredient
ADHD Drugs	Amphetamine aspartate, Amphetamine sulfate, Dextroamphetamine saccharate, Dextroamphetamine sulfate[a]
ADHD Drugs	Atomoxetine hydrochloride
ADHD Drugs	Clonidine
ADHD Drugs	Dexmethylphenidate hydrochloride
ADHD Drugs	Dextroamphetamine sulfate
ADHD Drugs	Guanfacine hydrochloride
ADHD Drugs	Lisdexamfetamine dimesylate
ADHD Drugs	Methamphetamine
ADHD Drugs	Methylphenidate hydrochloride
ADHD Drugs	Pemoline
Anti-anxiety	Alprazolam
Anti-anxiety	Buspirone hydrochloride
Anti-anxiety	Chlordiazepoxide hydrochloride
Anti-anxiety	Clonazepam
Anti-anxiety	Clorazepate dipotassium
Anti-anxiety	Diazepam
Anti-anxiety	Diphenhydramine hydrochloride
Anti-anxiety	Hydroxyzine
Anti-anxiety	Lorazepam
Anti-anxiety	Meprobamate
Anti-anxiety	Oxazepam
Anti-anxiety	Prazosin hydrochloride
Anti-anxiety	Propranolol hydrochloride
Anti-anxiety	Quazepam
Anticonvulsant	Carbamazepine
Anticonvulsant	Divalproex sodium
Anticonvulsant	Gabapentin
Anticonvulsant	Lamotrigine
Anticonvulsant	Oxcarbazepine

Type of psychotropic drug	Psychotropic drug ingredient
Anticonvulsant	Topiramate
Anticonvulsant	Valproate sodium
Anticonvulsant	Valproic acid
Antidepressants	Amitriptyline hydrochloride
Antidepressants	Amoxapine
Antidepressants	Bupropion hydrochloride
Antidepressants	Citalopram hydrobromide
Antidepressants	Clomipramine hydrochloride
Antidepressants	Desipramine hydrochloride
Antidepressants	Desvenlafaxine succinate
Antidepressants	Doxepin hydrochloride
Antidepressants	Duloxetine hydrochloride
Antidepressants	Escitalopram oxalate
Antidepressants	Fluoxetine hydrochloride
Antidepressants	Fluvoxamine maleate
Antidepressants	Imipramine
Antidepressants	Isocarboxazid
Antidepressants	Maprotiline hydrochloride
Antidepressants	Mirtazapine
Antidepressants	Nefazodone hydrochloride
Antidepressants	Nortriptyline hydrochloride
Antidepressants	Paroxetine
Antidepressants	Phenelzine sulfate
Antidepressants	Protriptyline hydrochloride
Antidepressants	Selegiline
Antidepressants	Sertraline hydrochloride
Antidepressants	Tranylcypromine sulfate
Antidepressants	Trazodone hydrochloride
Antidepressants	Trimipramine maleate
Antidepressants	Venlafaxine
Anti-enuretic	Desmopressin acetate
Antiparkinson	Amantadine hydrochloride
Antiparkinson	Benztropine mesylate
Antiparkinson	Trihexyphenidyl hydrochloride
Antipsychotics	Aripiprazole
Antipsychotics	Chlorpromazine
Antipsychotics	Clozapine
Antipsychotics	Droperidol
Antipsychotics	Fluphenazine
Antipsychotics	Haloperidol
Antipsychotics	Loxapine
Antipsychotics	Mesoridazine besylate
Antipsychotics	Molindone hydrochloride
Antipsychotics	Olanzapine
Antipsychotics	Paliperidone

Table 8. (Continued)

Type of psychotropic drug	Psychotropic drug ingredient
Antipsychotics	Perphenazine
Antipsychotics	Pimozide
Antipsychotics	Quetiapine fumarate
Antipsychotics	Risperidone
Antipsychotics	Thioridazine
Antipsychotics	Thiothixene
Antipsychotics	Trifluoperazine hydrochloride
Antipsychotics	Ziprasidone
Combination anti-anxiety and antidepressant	Amitriptyline and Chlordiazepoxide
Combination antipsychotic and antidepressant	Amitriptyline and Perphenazine
Combination antipsychotic and antidepressant	Olanzapine and Fluoxetine hydrochloride
Hypnotic	Estazolam
Hypnotic	Eszopiclone
Hypnotic	Flurazepam hydrochloride
Hypnotic	Midazolam hydrochloride
Hypnotic	Ramelteon
Hypnotic	Temazepam
Hypnotic	Triazolam
Hypnotic	Zaleplon
Hypnotic	Zolpidem tartrate
Mood stabilizer	Lithium
Sleep aid	Melatonin

Source: GAO.

[a] Amphetamine aspartate, amphetamine sulfate, dextroamphetamine saccharate, and dextroamphetamine sulfate are medications indicated for treatment of ADHD and, as such, were considered as a single ingredient for purposes of our review.

APPENDIX IV. RATES OF PSYCHOTROPIC PRESCRIPTION USAGE BY LENGTH OF TIME IN MEDICAID FEE-FOR-SERVICE

This appendix presents detailed information on rates of psychotropic prescriptions by the length of time a child was in a Medicaid fee-forservice program. In Michigan, Oregon, and Texas, psychotropic prescriptions were always covered by a fee-for-service program; in Florida and Massachusetts, prescriptions were covered by either Medicaid fee-for-service or a managed care program. In our analysis of Florida's Medicaid program, we found that children in foster care for 30 days or more averaged 7.47 months of fee-for-service coverage compared to 5.02 months for nonfoster children. To determine the impact of different lengths of time in fee-for-service on rates of psychotropic prescription usage, we conducted an analysis that adjusted for length of time in fee-for-service in Florida. Table 9 shows the rates of psychotropic prescription usage for children under 18 by length of time in fee-for-service.

Table 9. Rates of Psychotropic Prescriptions by Length of Medicaid Fee-for-service Coverage in Florida during 2008

Length of time in Medicaid fee-for-service	Foster children age 0-17, in care for 30 or more days		Nonfoster children age 0-17		Ratio of percentage with 1 or more psychotropic prescriptions of foster to nonfoster children
	Population	Percentage with 1 or more psychotropic prescription	Population	Percentage with 1 or more psychotropic prescription	
3-5 months	899	6.7	87,161	2.8	2.4
6-8 months	1,338	11.8	71,505	4.1	2.9
9-12 months	16,817	24.1	456,219	11.0	2.2
1-12 months	19,484	22.0	686,103	8.2	2.7
Children enrolled in Medicaid fee-for -service or managed care organization during 2008	32,806		1,526,020		

Source: GAO analysis of Florida Medicaid and foster care data.

APPENDIX V. ADDITIONAL DATA ON CHILDREN WITH PRESCRIPTIONS OF AT LEAST ONE PSYCHOTROPIC DRUG

This appendix presents detailed information on rates of foster and nonfoster children prescribed at least one psychotropic drug in the five states during 2008. In the tables below, rates for foster and nonfoster children can be compared within the same state and the ratio of prescriptions to foster children to prescriptions to nonfoster children can be compared across states. However, prescription rates cannot be compared across states. Percentages and ratios are rounded to the nearest tenth, and therefore the reported ratio may be slightly different than the ratio of the rounded percentages.

Table 10. Rates of Psychotropic Prescriptions in Florida during 2008 by Age of Child and Foster Care Status

Age	Foster children		Nonfoster children		Ratio of foster to nonfoster children
	Number	Percent	Number	Percentage	
Children 0-17 (Under18)	4,281	22.0	56,408	8.2	2.7
Children 13-17	2,093	36.8	17,549	11.9	3.1
Children 6-12	1,758	31.2	28,690	12.3	2.5
Children 0-5 (Under 6)	430	5.3	10,169	3.3	1.6

Source: GAO analysis of Florida Medicaid and foster care data.

Table 11. Rates of Psychotropic Prescriptions in Massachusetts during 2008 by Age of Child and Foster Care Status

Age	Foster children		Nonfoster children		Ratio of foster to nonfoster children
	Number	Percentage	Number	Percentage	
Children 0-17 (Under 18)	3,814	39.1	22,041	10.2	3.8
Children 13-17	2,599	53.4	10,265	14.7	3.6
Children 6-12	1,095	44.8	10,455	12.1	3.7
Children 0-5 (Under 6)	120	4.9	1,321	2.2	2.2

Source: GAO analysis of Massachusetts Medicaid and foster care data.

Table 12. Rates of Psychotropic Prescriptions in Michigan during 2008 by Age of Child and Foster Care Status

Age	Foster children		Nonfoster children		Ratio of foster to nonfoster children
	Number	Percentage	Number	Percentage	
Children 0-17 (Under 18)	4,360	21.0	74,188	7.9	2.7
Children 13-17	2,220	35.0	30,118	13.1	2.7
Children 6-12	1,802	26.7	39,917	11.5	2.3
Children 0-5 (Under 6)	338	4.4	4,153	1.1	3.8

Source: GAO analysis of Michigan Medicaid and foster care data.

Table 13. Rates of Psychotropic Prescriptions in Oregon during 2008 by Age of Child and Foster Care Status

Age	Foster children		Nonfoster children		Ratio of foster to nonfoster children
	Number	Percentage	Number	Percentage	
Children 0-17 (Under 18)	2,119	19.7	11,731	4.8	4.1
Children 13-17	1,177	43.3	5,991	12.0	3.6
Children 6-12	831	23.4	5,022	6.2	3.8
Children 0-5 (Under 6)	111	2.5	718	0.6	3.9

Source: GAO analysis of Oregon Medicaid and foster care data.

Table 14. Rates of Psychotropic Prescriptions in Texas during 2008 by Age of Child and Foster Care Status

Age	Foster children		Nonfoster children		Ratio of foster to nonfoster children
	Number	Percentage	Number	Percentage	
Children 0-17 (Under 18)	11,699	32.2	185,329	7.1	4.5
Children 13-17	4,740	58.2	53,142	11.4	5.1
Children 6-12	5,488	45.8	93,466	10.6	4.3
Children 0-5 (Under 6)	1,471	9.1	38,721	3.1	2.9

Source: GAO analysis of Texas Medicaid and foster care data.

APPENDIX VI. ADDITIONAL DATA ON CONCOMITANT PRESCRIPTIONS

This appendix presents detailed information on rates of psychotropic drugs prescribed concomitantly to foster and nonfoster children under 18 years old during 2008. We considered two or more drugs with unique active ingredients to be prescribed concomitantly if each prescription was filled with a 3-month overlap, defined as 84 days to account for prescriptions that are filled late and 28-day prescriptions. We did not count two drugs with the same active ingredient such as a brand name drug and its generic equivalent. We did count combination drugs, which have two active ingredients in a single dose, as concomitant prescriptions.[58]

In the tables below, rates for foster and nonfoster children can be compared within the same state and the ratio of prescriptions to foster children to prescriptions to nonfoster children can be compared across states. However, prescription rates cannot be compared across states. Percentages and ratios are rounded to the nearest tenth, and therefore the reported ratio may be slightly different than the ratio of the rounded percentages.

Table 15. Rates of Concomitant Psychotropic Prescriptions in Florida during 2008 by Number of Drugs

Medications prescribed concomitantly	Foster children		Nonfoster children		Ratio of foster to nonfoster children
	Number	Percentage	Number	Percentage	
Children 0-17					
1 (combination drug)	-	0.0	-	0.0	-
2	715	3.7	4,689	0.7	5.4
3	323	1.7	1,863	0.3	6.1
4	93	0.5	564	0.1	5.8
5	18	0.1	137	0.0	4.6
6	<10	0.0	37	0.0	3.8
7	-	0.0	11	0.0	-
8	-	0.0	<10	0.0	-
9	-	0.0	<10	0.0	-
10	-	0.0	-	0.0	-
Total	**>1149**	**5.9**	**>7,301**	**1.1**	**5.6**

Table 15. (Continued)

Medications prescribed concomitantly	Foster children		Nonfoster children		Ratio of foster to nonfoster children
	Number	Percentage	Number	Percentage	
Children 13-17					
1 (combination drug)	-	0.0	-	0.0	-
2	376	6.6	1,727	1.2	5.6
3	182	3.2	819	0.6	5.7
4	55	1.0	307	0.2	4.6
5	11	0.2	74	0.1	3.8
6	<10	0.0	22	0.0	2.4
7	-	0.0	<10	0.0	-
8	-	0.0	-	0.0	-
9	-	0.0	<10	0.0	-
10	-	0.0	-	0.0	-
Total	**>624**	**11.0**	**>2,949**	**2.0**	**5.5**
Children 6-12					
1 (combination drug)	-	0.0	-	0.0	-
2	315	5.6	2,680	1.1	4.9
3	138	2.4	988	0.4	5.8
4	37	0.7	249	0.1	6.2
5	<10	0.1	62	0.0	4.7
6	<10	0.0	15	0.0	5.5
7	-	0.0	<10	0.0	-
8	-	0.0	<10	0.0	-
9	-	0.0	-	0.0	-
10	-	0.0	-	0.0	-
Total	**>490**	**8.9**	**>3994**	**1.7**	**5.2**
Children 0-5					
1 (combination drug)	-	0.0	-	0.0	-
2	24	0.3	282	0.1	3.2
3	<10	0.0	56	0.0	2.0
4	<10	0.0	<10	0.0	4.7
5	-	0.0	<10	0.0	-
Total	**>24**	**0.3**	**>338**	**0.1**	**3.0**

Source: GAO analysis of Florida Medicaid and foster care data.

Note: Percentages are rounded to the nearest tenth.

Table 16. Rates of Concomitant Psychotropic Prescriptions in Massachusetts during 2008 by Number of Drugs

Medications prescribed concomitantly	Foster children		Nonfoster children		Ratio of foster to nonfoster children
	Number	Percentage	Number	Percentage	
Children 0-17					
1 (combination drug)	-	0.0	-	0.0	-
2	711	7.3	2,586	1.2	6.1
3	558	5.7	1,171	0.5	10.6
4	249	2.5	430	0.2	12.8
5	97	1.0	118	0.1	18.2
6	26	0.3	31	0.0	18.6
7	<10	0.1	<10	0.0	12.3
8	<10	0.0	-	0.0	-
9	-	0.0	-	0.0	-
10	-	0.0	<10	0.0	-
Total	**>1641**	**16.9**	**>4,336**	**2.0**	**8.4**
Children 13-17					
1 (combination drug)	-	0.0	-	0.0	-
2	473	9.7	1,103	1.6	6.2
3	368	7.6	588	0.8	9.0
4	176	3.6	258	0.4	9.8
5	76	1.6	84	0.1	13.0
6	19	0.4	22	0.0	12.4
7	<10	0.1	<10	0.0	9.0
8	<10	0.0	-	0.0	-
9	-	0.0	-	0.0	-
10	-	0.0	<10	0.0	-
Total	**>1,112**	**23.0**	**>2,055**	**3.0**	**7.8**
Children 6-12					
1 (combination drug)	-	0.0	-	0.0	-
2	228	9.3	1,413	1.6	5.7
3	184	7.5	563	0.7	11.5
4	73	3.0	170	0.2	15.1
5	21	0.9	34	0.0	21.8
6	<10	0.3	<10	0.0	27.4
7	-	0.0	<10	0.0	-
8	-	0.0	-	0.0	-
9	-	0.0	-	0.0	-
10	-	0.0	-	0.0	-
Total	**>506**	**21.0**	**>2,180**	**2.5**	**8.3**

Medications prescribed concomitantly	Foster children		Nonfoster children		Ratio of foster to nonfoster children
	Number	Percentage	Number	Percentage	
Children 0-5					
1 (combination drug)	-	0.0	-	0.0	-
2	10	0.4	70	0.1	3.5
3	<10	0.2	20	0.0	7.4
4	-	0.0	<10	0.0	-
5	-	0.0	-	0.0	-
Total	**>10**	**0.7**	**>90**	**0.2**	**4.3**

Source: GAO analysis of Massachusetts Medicaid and foster care data.
Note: Percentages are rounded to the nearest tenth.

Table 17. Rates of Concomitant Psychotropic Prescriptions in Michigan during 2008 by Number of Drugs

Medications prescribed concomitantly	Foster children		Nonfoster children		Ratio of foster to nonfoster children
	Number	Percentage	Number	Percentage	
Children 0-17					
1(combination drug)	-	0.0	<10	0.0	-
2	620	3.0	5,659	0.6	5.0
3	332	1.6	1,951	0.2	7.7
4	134	0.6	608	0.1	10.0
5	50	0.2	152	0.0	14.9
6	10	0.0	34	0.0	13.3
7	<10	0.0	10	0.0	4.5
8	-	0.0	<10	0.0	-

Table 17. (Continued)

Medications prescribed concomitantly	Foster children		Nonfoster children		Ratio of foster to nonfoster children
	Number	Percentage	Number	Percentage	
9	-	0.0	-	0.0	-
10	-	0.0	-	0.0	-
Total	**>1,146**	**5.5**	**>8,414**	**0.9**	**6.2**
Children 13-17					
1(combination drug)	-	0.0	<10	0.0	-
2	367	5.8	2,435	1.1	5.5
3	234	3.7	1,045	0.5	8.1
4	97	1.5	378	0.2	9.3
5	38	0.6	95	0.0	14.5
6	<10	0.1	25	0.0	13.1
7	<10	0.0	<10	0.0	6.1
8	-	0.0	<10	0.0	-
9	-	0.0	-	0.0	-
10	-	0.0	-	0.0	-
Total	**>736**	**11.8**	**>3,978**	**1.7**	**6.8**
Children 6-12					
1(combination drug)	-	0.0	-	0.0	-
2	236	3.5	3,044	0.9	4.0
3	95	1.4	877	0.3	5.6
4	37	0.5	228	0.1	8.3
5	12	0.2	57	0.0	10.8
6	<10	0.0	<10	0.0	5.7
7	-	0.0	<10	0.0	-
8	-	0.0	-	0.0	-
9	-	0.0	-	0.0	-
10	-	0.0	-	0.0	-
Total	**>380**	**5.6**	**>4,206**	**1.2**	**4.6**
Children 0-5					
1 (combination drug)	-	0.0	-	0.0	-
2	17	0.2	180	0.0	4.5
3	<10	0.0	29	0.0	4.9
4	-	0.0	<10	0.0	-
5	-	0.0	-	0.0	-
Total	**>17**	**0.3**	**>209**	**0.1**	**4.5**

Source: GAO analysis of Michigan Medicaid and foster care data.

Note: Percentages are rounded to the nearest tenth.

Table 18. Rates of Concomitant Psychotropic Prescriptions in Oregon during 2008 by Number of Drugs

Medications prescribed concomitantly	Foster children		Nonfoster children		Ratio of foster to nonfoster children
	Number	Percentage	Number	Percentage	
Children 0-17					
1 (combination drug)	-	0.0	<10	0.0	-
2	330	3.1	980	0.4	7.6
3	131	1.2	317	0.1	9.4
4	31	0.3	91	0.0	7.7
5	11	0.1	19	0.0	13.1
6	<10	0.0	<10	0.0	4.5
7	<10	0.0	-	0.0	-
8	-	0.0	-	0.0	-
9	-	0.0	-	0.0	-
10	-	0.0	-	0.0	-
Total	**>503**	**4.7**	**>1,407**	**0.6**	**8.1**
Children 13-17					
1 (combination drug)	-	0.0	<10	0.0	-
2	214	7.9	488	1.0	8.0
3	90	3.3	172	0.3	9.6
4	24	0.9	58	0.1	7.6
5	<10	0.3	<10	0.0	20.9
6	-	0.0	<10	0.0	-
7	<10	0.1	-	0.0	-
8	-	0.0	-	0.0	-
9	-	0.0	-	0.0	-
10	-	0.0	-	0.0	-
Total	**>328**	**12.4**	**>718**	**1.5**	**8.5**
Children 6-12					
1 (combination drug)	-	0.0	-	0.0	-
2	109	3.1	473	0.6	5.3
3	40	1.1	137	0.2	6.7
4	<10	0.2	33	0.0	4.9
5	<10	0.1	12	0.0	5.8
6	<10	0.0	<10	0.0	7.7
7	-	0.0	-	0.0	-
8	-	0.0	-	0.0	-
9	-	0.0	-	0.0	-
10	-	0.0	-	0.0	-
Total	**>149**	**4.5**	**>655**	**0.8**	**5.6**

Table 18. (Continued).

Medications prescribed concomitantly	Foster children		Nonfoster children		Ratio of foster to nonfoster children
	Number	Percentage	Number	Percentage	
Children 0-5					
1 (combination drug)	-	0.0	-	0.0	-
2	<10	0.2	19	0.0	9.3
3	<10	0.0	<10	0.0	3.1
4	-	0.0	-	0.0	-
5	-	0.0	-	0.0	-
Total	**>0**	**0.2**	**>19**	**0.0**	**7.4**

Source: GAO analysis of Oregon Medicaid and foster care data.

Note: Percentages are rounded to the nearest tenth.

Table 19. Rates of Concomitant Psychotropic Prescriptions in Texas during 2008 by Number of Drugs

Medications prescribed concomitantly	Foster children		Nonfoster children		Ratio of foster to nonfoster children
	Number	Percentage	Number	Percentage	
Children 0-17					
1(combination drug)	<10	0.0	14	0.0	5.1
2	2,483	6.8	11,002	0.4	16.2
3	1,672	4.6	4,518	0.2	26.5
4	839	2.3	1,549	0.1	38.8
5	301	0.8	415	0.0	52.0
6	60	0.2	126	0.0	34.1
7	18	0.0	21	0.0	61.4
8	<10	0.0	10	0.0	14.3
9	<10	0.0	-	0.0	-
10	-	0.0	<10	0.0	-
Total	**>5,373**	**14.8**	**>17,655**	**0.7**	**21.8**
Children 13-17					
1 (combination drug)	-	0.0	13	0.0	-
2	1,044	12.8	3,652	0.8	16.4
3	758	9.3	1,792	0.4	24.3
4	422	5.2	692	0.1	35.0
5	128	1.6	206	0.0	35.7

Table 19. (Continued)

Medications prescribed concomitantly	Foster children		Nonfoster children		Ratio of foster to nonfoster children
	Number	Percentage	Number	Percentage	
6	38	0.5	78	0.0	28.0
7	14	0.2	15	0.0	53.6
8	<10	0.0	<10	0.0	11.5
9	-	0.0	-	0.0	-
10	-	0.0	<10	0.0	-
Total	**>2,404**	**29.5**	**>6,448**	**1.4**	**21.4**
Children 6-12					
1 (combination drug)	<10	0.0	<10	0.0	73.3
2	1,245	10.4	6,504	0.7	14.0
3	820	6.8	2,552	0.3	23.6
4	403	3.4	822	0.1	36.0
5	171	1.4	206	0.0	60.9
6	22	0.2	48	0.0	33.6
7	<10	0.0	<10	0.0	48.9
8	<10	0.0	<10	0.0	14.7
9	<10	0.0	-	0.0	-
10	-	0.0	<10	0.0	-
Total	**>2,661**	**22.3**	**>10,132**	**1.2**	**19.3**
Children 0-5					
1 (combination drug)	-	0.0	-	0.0	-
2	194	1.2	846	0.1	17.8
3	94	0.6	174	0.0	41.9
4	14	0.1	35	0.0	31.0
5	<10	0.0	<10	0.0	51.7
Total	**>302**	**1.9**	**>1,055**	**0.1**	**22.3**

Source: GAO analysis of Texas Medicaid and foster care data.

Note: Percentages are rounded to the nearest tenth.

Appendix VII. Additional Data on Psychotropic Drug Prescriptions Exceeding Maximum Recommended Doses

This appendix presents detailed information on rates of psychotropic drugs prescribed for foster and nonfoster children that exceeded the maximum dose for the child's age cited in the Texas Utilization Parameters, which includes doses based on information in the FDA- approved drug label and published in medical literature for the child's age. Based on these parameters, we also analyzed prescriptions where there was no FDA-approved dose or published dose in medical literature for the child's age. Finally, for those prescriptions that had no FDA-approved doses for the child's age, we determined whether the prescription dosage exceeded the next most relevant standard: dosages published in medical literature for the same age group, dosages published in medical literature for an older age group, or the FDA-approved dose for an older age group or similar version of the same drug. These dosages were drawn from the Texas Utilization Parameters or, in limited cases, FDA-approved drug labels.

In the tables below, rates for foster and nonfoster children can be compared within the same state and the ratio of prescriptions to foster children to prescriptions to nonfoster children can be compared across states. However, prescription rates cannot be compared across states. Percentages and ratios are rounded to the nearest tenth, and therefore the reported ratio may be slightly different than the ratio of the rounded percentages.

Table 20. Rates of Children Prescribed Psychotropic Drugs Outside FDA-Approved Doses or Standards Published in Medical Literature in Florida during 2008

Category	Foster		Nonfoster		Ratio of foster to nonfoster children
	Number	Percentage	Number	Percentage	
Prescription exceeding FDA maximum dose for age group	292	1.5	3,005	0.4	3.4
Prescription exceeding maximum dose published in medical literature for age group	423	2.2	3,566	0.5	4.2
Prescription with no FDA-approved dose for child's age, exceeding dosages for the next most relevant standard	101	0.5	586	0.1	6.1
Prescription for medication with no FDA-approved dose for age group	1,628	8.4	15,282	2.2	3.8
Prescription for medication with no published dose in medical literature for age group	71	0.4	828	0.1	3.0

Source: GAO analysis of Florida Medicaid and foster care data.

Note: The data contained for each category in this table are not mutually exclusive.

Table 21. Rates of Children Prescribed Psychotropic Drugs Outside FDA-Approved Doses or Standards Published in Medical Literature in Massachusetts during 2008

Category	Foster		Nonfoster		Ratio of foster to nonfoster children
	Number	Percentage	Number	Percentage	
Prescription exceeding FDA maximum dose for age group	216	2.2	1,214	0.6	3.9
Prescription exceeding maximum dose published in medical literature for age group	367	3.8	1,590	0.7	5.1
Prescription with no FDA-approved dose for child's age, exceeding dosages for the next most relevant standard	116	1.2	336	0.2	7.7
Prescription for medication with no FDA-approved dose for age group	2,199	22.5	8,287	3.8	5.9
Prescription for medication with no published dose in medical literature for age group	88	0.9	433	0.2	4.5

Source: GAO analysis of Massachusetts Medicaid and foster care data.

Note: The data contained for each category in this table are not mutually exclusive.

Table 22. Rates of Children Prescribed Psychotropic Drugs Outside FDA-Approved Doses or Standards Published in Medical Literature in Michigan during 2008

Category	Foster		Nonfoster		Ratio of foster to Nonfoster children
	Number	Percentage	Number	Percentage	
Prescription exceeding FDA maximum dose for age group	346	1.7	4,592	0.5	3.4
Prescription exceeding maximum dose published in medical literature for age group	412	2.0	4,660	0.5	4.0
Prescription with no FDA-approved dose for child's age, exceeding dosages for the next most relevant standard	70	0.3	492	0.1	6.4
Prescription for medication with no FDA-approved dose for age group	1,411	6.8	14,026	1.5	4.6
Prescription for medication with no published dose in medical literature for age group	186	0.9	1,750	0.2	4.8

Source: GAO analysis of Michigan Medicaid and foster care data.

Note: The data contained for each category in this table are not mutually exclusive.

Table 23. Rates of Children Prescribed Psychotropic Drugs Outside FDA-Approved Doses or Standards Published in Medical Literature in Oregon during 2008

Category	Foster		Nonfoster		Ratio of foster to Nonfoster children
	Number	Percentage	Number	Percentage	
Prescription exceeding FDA maximum dose for age group	121	1.1	399	0.2	6.9
Prescription exceeding maximum dose pu- blished in medical literature for age group	180	1.7	539	0.2	7.6
Prescription with no FDA-approved dose for child's age, exceeding dosages for the next most relevant standard	43	0.4	115	0.1	8.5
Prescription for medication with no FDA-approved dose for age group	726	6.8	3,063	1.3	5.4
Prescription for medication with no published dose in medical literature for age group	61	0.6	334	0.1	4.1

Source: GAO analysis of Oregon Medicaid and foster care data.

Note: The data contained for each category in this table are not mutually exclusive.

Table 24. Rates of Children Prescribed Psychotropic Drugs Outside FDA-Approved Doses or Standards Published in Medical Literature in Texas during 2008

Category	Foster		Nonfoster		Ratio of foster to Nonfoster children
	Number	Percentage	Number	Percentage	
Prescription exceeding FDA maximum dose for age group	1,190	3.3	9,590	0.4	8.9
Prescription exceeding maximum dose published in medical literature for age group	1,773	4.9	11,033	0.4	11.5
Prescription with no FDA-approved dose for child's age, exceeding dosages for the next most relevant standard	554	1.5	1,849	0.1	21.5
Prescription for medication with no FDA-approved dose for age group	6,060	16.7	42,328	1.6	10.3
Prescription for medication with no published dose in medical literature for age group	861	2.4	4,232	0.2	14.6

Source: GAO analysis of Texas Medicaid and foster care data.

Note: The data contained for each category in this table are not mutually exclusive.

APPENDIX VIII. ADDITIONAL DATA ON PSYCHOTROPIC PRESCRIPTIONS TO CHILDREN UNDER 1 YEAR OLD

This appendix presents detailed information on psychotropic prescriptions to children under 1 year old in five selected states.

Table 25. Prescriptions of Psychotropic Drugs to Foster and Nonfoster Children Age 0-1 in Five Selected States

Category	Ingredient	Foster children		Nonfoster children	
		Children	Pres-criptions	Children	Pres-criptions
ADHD Drugs	Clonidine	<10	17	22	46
	Guanfacine hydrochloride	0	0	<10	<10
	Amphetamine aspartate, amphetamine sulfate, dextroamphetamine saccharate, dextroampheta-mine sulfate	0	0	<10	<10
	Lisdexamfetamine dimesylate	0	0	<10	<10
	Methylphenidate hydrochloride	0	0	<10	12
	Subtotal	<10	17	40	76
Anti-anxiety	Diphenhydramine hydrochloride (antihistamine)	<10	<10	49	54
	Hydroxyzine (antihistamine)	52	70	3,408	4,240
	Alprazolam (benzodiazepine)	0	0	14	32
	Clonazepam (benzodiazepine)	<10	18	69	219
	Clorazepate dipotassium (benzodiazepine)	<10	14	<10	<10
	Diazepam (benzodiazepine)	<10	22	95	220
	Lorazepam (benzodiazepine)	<10	15	91	127
	Buspirone hydrochloride	0	0	<10	<10
	Subtotal	74	142	3,730	4,899
Antidepressants	Bupropion hydrochloride	<10	<10	<10	<10
	Trazodone hydrochloride	0	0	<10	16
	Venlafaxine	0	0	<10	<10
	Citalopram hydrobromide	0	0	<10	12
	Escitalopram oxalate	<10	<10	11	24
	Fluoxetine hydrochloride	0	0	<10	<10
	Paroxetine	0	0	<10	<10
	Sertraline hydrochloride	0	0	12	16
	Amitriptyline hydrochloride	<10	<10	0	0
	Doxepin hydrochloride	<10	<10	0	0
	Subtotal	<10	18	49	87

Table 25. (Continued)

Category	Ingredient	Foster children		Nonfoster children	
		Children	Pres-criptions	Children	Pres-criptions
Antipsychotics	Aripiprazole	0	0	<10	<10
	Olanzapine	0	0	<10	<10
	Quetiapine fumarate	<10	<10	<10	<10
	Risperidone	0	0	<10	<10
	Ziprasidone	0	0	<10	<10
	Subtotal	<10	<10	12	15
Hypnotic	Triazolam	0	0	<10	<10
	Zolpidem tartrate	0	0	<10	<10
	Subtotal	0	0	<10	<10
Mood stabilizer	Lithium	0	0	<10	<10
Total[a]		**85**	**182**	**3,836**	**5,083**

Source: GAO analysis of state Medicaid and foster care data.

[a] Note: These subtotals and total differ from those in table 2 because children prescribed multiple ingredients from the same category of drug are listed once for each ingredient in the table above, and therefore may be counted multiple times per category. In table 2, children are counted only once per category of drug.

APPENDIX IX. ADDITIONAL DATA ON PSYCHOTROPIC DRUGS WITH GAPS IN PRESCRIPTIONS OF 7 TO 29 DAYS

This appendix presents detailed information on psychotropic drugs prescribed for foster and nonfoster children with gaps in prescriptions of 7-29 days. While children in foster care had a higher rate of three or more gaps in prescriptions for a single active ingredient in all states, other differences between gaps in prescriptions for foster and nonfoster children varied by state.

In the tables below, rates for foster and nonfoster children can be compared within the same state. However, prescription rates cannot be compared across states. Since we used both primary and secondary lists in our gaps analysis, the number of foster and nonfoster children prescribed a psychotropic drug is slightly higher than reported in our overall prescription rates, which were based on primary drugs only.

Table 26. Rates of Psychotropic Drugs with Three or More Gaps of 7-29 Days in Prescriptions to Foster and Nonfoster Children in Florida during 2008

Age	Number of children who had three or more gaps in drug claims		Percentage of foster or nonfoster children who had three or more gaps in drug claims		Percentage of foster or nonfoster children prescribed a psychotropic drug who had three or more gaps in drug claims	
	Foster Children	Non-foster children	Foster children	Non-foster children	Foster children	Non-foster children
0-17	355	7,381	1.8	1.1	7.8	12.1
13-17	159	2,379	2.8	1.6	7.2	12.6
6-12	167	4,489	3.0	1.9	9.1	14.5
0-5	29	513	0.4	0.2	5.9	4.6

Source: GAO analysis of Florida Medicaid and foster care data.

Table 27. Average Gaps of 7-29 Days in Psychotropic Drug Prescriptions to Foster and Nonfoster Children in Florida during 2008

Age	Category	Children in Medicaid with a psychotropic prescription (including those with or without a gap in prescriptions)		Children in Medicaid with at least one gap in psychotropic drug prescriptions	
		Foster	Nonfoster	Foster	Nonfoster
0-17	Average number of gaps per child	1.09	1.18	1.59	1.85
	Average length of gaps per child (days)	9.64	9.63	13.98	15.01
13-17	Average number of gaps per child	1.15	1.33	1.57	1.82
	Average length of gaps per child (days)	10.35	11.03	14.05	15.04
6-12	Average number of gaps per child	1.13	1.35	1.60	1.88
	Average length of gaps per child (days)	9.82	10.72	13.89	14.94
0-5	Average number of gaps per child	0.68	0.48	1.65	1.74
	Average length of gaps per child (days)	5.75	4.24	14.01	15.28

Source: GAO analysis of Florida Medicaid and foster care data.

Table 28. Rates of Psychotropic Drugs with Three or More Gaps of 7-29 Days in Prescriptions to Foster and Nonfoster Children in Massachusetts during 2008

Age	Number of children who had three or more gaps in drug claims		Percentage of foster or nonfoster children who had three or more gaps in drug claims		Percentage of foster or nonfoster children prescribed a psychotropic drug who had three or more gaps in drug claims	
	Foster Children	Nonfoster children	Foster children	Nonfoster children	Foster children	Nonfoster children
0-17	330	3,825	3.4	1.8	8.4	16.4
13-17	210	1,769	4.3	2.5	7.8	16.4
6-12	112	1,954	4.6	2.3	9.9	17.6
0-5	<10	102	0.3	0.2	6.2	6.9

Source: GAO analysis of Massachusetts Medicaid and foster care data.

Table 29. Average Gaps of 7-29 Days in Psychotropic Drug Prescriptions to Foster and Nonfoster Children in Massachusetts during 2008

Age	Category	Children in Medicaid with a psychotropic prescription (including those with or without a gap in prescriptions)		Children in Medicaid with at least one gap in psychotropic drug prescriptions	
		Foster	Nonfoster	Foster	Nonfoster
0-17	Average number of gaps per child	1.14	1.55	1.56	1.94
	Average length of gaps per child (days)	10.57	11.90	14.37	14.87
13-17	Average number of gaps per child	1.14	1.62	1.54	1.94
	Average length of gaps per child (days)	10.65	12.43	14.42	14.88
6-12	Average number of gaps per child	1.22	1.60	1.58	1.95
	Average length of gaps per child (days)	11.00	12.14	14.27	14.84
0-5	Average number of gaps per child	0.55	0.74	1.50	1.79
	Average length of gaps per child (days)	5.14	6.30	13.93	15.18

Source: GAO analysis of Massachusetts Medicaid and foster care data.

Table 30. Rates of Psychotropic Drugs with Three or More Gaps of 7-29 Days in Prescriptions to Foster and Nonfoster Children in Michigan during 2008

Age	Number of children who had three or more gaps in drug claims		Percentage of foster or nonfoster children who had three or more gaps in drug claims		Percentage of foster or nonfoster children prescribed a psychotropic drug who had three or more gaps in drug claims	
	Foster children	Nonfoster children	Foster children	Nonfoster children	Foster children	Nonfoster children
0-17	360	8,903	1.7	0.9	7.9	11.3
13-17	165	3,459	2.6	1.5	7.2	10.8
6-12	174	5,122	2.6	1.5	9.3	12.2
0-5	21	322	0.3	0.1	5.6	6.4

Source: GAO analysis of Michigan Medicaid and foster care data.

Table 31. Average Gaps of 7-29 Days in Psychotropic Drug Prescriptions to Foster and Nonfoster Children in Michigan during 2008

Age	Category	Children in Medicaid with a psychotropic prescription (including those with or without a gap in prescriptions)		Children in Medicaid with at least one gap in psychotropic drug prescriptions	
		Foster	Nonfoster	Foster	Nonfoster
0-17	Average number of gaps per child	1.10	1.14	1.60	1.76
	Average length of gaps per child (days)	10.03	9.61	14.55	14.85
13-17	Average number of gaps per child	1.14	1.18	1.55	1.74
	Average length of gaps per child (days)	10.67	10.16	14.47	14.96
6-12	Average number of gaps per child	1.15	1.17	1.67	1.79
	Average length of gaps per child (days)	9.99	9.67	14.53	14.76
0-5	Average number of gaps per child	0.67	0.65	1.64	1.71
	Average length of gaps per child (days)	6.34	5.68	15.61	14.97

Source: GAO analysis of Michigan Medicaid and foster care data.

Table 32. Rates of Psychotropic Drugs with Three or More Gaps of 7-29 Days in Prescriptions to Foster and Nonfoster Children in Oregon during 2008

Age	Number of children who had three or more gaps in drug claims		Percentage of foster or nonfoster children who had three or more gaps in drug claims		Percentage of foster or nonfoster children prescribed a psychotropic drug who had three or more gaps in drug claims	
	Foster children	Nonfoster children	Foster children	Nonfoster children	Foster children	Nonfoster children
0-17	167	1,174	1.6	0.5	7.7	9.5
13-17	97	576	3.6	1.2	8.1	9.3
6-12	61	559	1.7	0.7	7.2	10.5
0-5	<10	39	0.2	0.0	7.1	4.7

Source: GAO analysis of Oregon Medicaid and foster care data.

Table 33. Average Gaps of 7-29 Days in Psychotropic Drug Prescriptions to Foster and Nonfoster Children in Oregon during 2008

Age	Category	Children in Medicaid with a psychotropic prescription (including those with or without a gap in prescriptions)		Children in Medicaid with at least one gap in psychotropic drug prescriptions	
		Foster	Nonfoster	Foster	Nonfoster
0-17	Average number of gaps per child	0.96	0.95	1.63	1.79
	Average length of gaps per child (days)	8.31	7.70	14.15	14.53
13-17	Average number of gaps per child	1.06	0.95	1.62	1.77
	Average length of gaps per child (days)	9.06	7.75	13.88	14.46
6-12	Average number of gaps per child	0.88	1.01	1.64	1.81
	Average length of gaps per child (days)	7.75	8.12	14.51	14.55
0-5	Average number of gaps per child	0.57	0.52	1.71	1.72
	Average length of gaps per child (days)	5.08	4.63	15.37	15.15

Source: GAO analysis of Oregon Medicaid and foster care data.

Table 34. Rates of Psychotropic Drugs with Three or More Gaps of 7-29 Days in Prescriptions to Foster and Nonfoster Children in Texas during 2008

Age	Number of children who had three or more gaps in drug claims		Percentage of foster or nonfoster children who had three or more gaps in drug claims		Percentage of foster or nonfoster children prescribed a psychotropic drug who had three or more gaps in drug claims	
	Foster children	Nonfoster children	Foster children	Nonfoster children	Foster children	Nonfoster children
0-17	798	17,512	2.2	0.7	6.6	8.6
13-17	336	5,185	4.1	1.1	7.0	9.1
6-12	373	10,935	3.1	1.2	6.6	10.8
0-5	89	1,392	0.5	0.1	5.6	3.2

Source: GAO analysis of Texas Medicaid and foster care data.

Table 35. Average Gaps of 7-29 Days in Psychotropic Drug Prescriptions to Foster and Nonfoster Children in Texas during 2008

Age	Category	Children in Medicaid with a psychotropic prescription (including those with or without a gap in prescriptions)		Children in Medicaid with at least one gap in psychotropic drug prescriptions	
		Foster	Nonfoster	Foster	Nonfoster
0-17	Average number of gaps per child	1.23	0.94	1.44	1.73
	Average length of gaps per child (days)	11.97	8.37	14.00	15.32
13-17	Average number of gaps per child	1.38	1.08	1.42	1.71
	Average length of gaps per child (days)	13.75	9.72	14.13	15.38
6-12	Average number of gaps per child	1.25	1.12	1.45	1.76
	Average length of gaps per child (days)	11.92	9.73	13.85	15.26
0-5	Average number of gaps per child	0.74	0.36	1.54	1.62
	Average length of gaps per child (days)	6.77	3.44	14.09	15.52

Source: GAO analysis of Texas Medicaid and foster care data.

APPENDIX X. SELECTED STATES' IMPLEMENTATION OF AACAP'S BEST PRINCIPLES GUIDELINES

This appendix compares in detail selected states' oversight of psychotropic drug prescriptions for foster children with the American Academy of Child and Adolescent Psychiatry (AACAP) Best Principles Guidelines. The processes were in place as of October 2011 unless otherwise noted. The tables are based on interviews and documentation provided by state Medicaid and foster care officials. With the exception of table 39, the information below was not tested to ensure these principles are implemented effectively.

Table 36. State Consent Laws and Policies Compared with AACAP Best Principle Guidelines

State	Extent	Description
AACAP guideline		**Identify the parties empowered to consent for psychotropic drug treatment for youth in state custody in a timely fashion [minimal].**
FL	Full	The parent or legal guardian can consent for psychotropic drug treatment, or the foster care agency may seek court authorization.
MD	Full	The parent, legal guardian, court-authorized foster care agency, or local social services director or designee can consent for psychotropic drug treatment.
MA	Full	For children in the care of the Massachusetts Department of Children and Families (DCF) through a voluntary placement agreement, only parents may consent to the use of antipsychotic drugs. For children in the custody of the Massachusetts DCF through a court order or through adoption surrender, court approval is required for the use of antipsychotic drugs in all non- emergency cases. According to agency officials, parents whose rights have not been terminated, caseworkers, or foster parents can provide consent for all other psychotropic medications.
MI	Full	For children in the care of the Michigan Department of Human Services (DHS) through a voluntary placement, or children who are temporary wards of the court, only parents or legal guardians may consent to the use of psychotropic drugs. For children who are permanent wards of the court, only the court may consent to the use of psychotropic drugs. For children who are permanent wards of the state, only the Michigan DHS may consent to the use of psychotropic drugs.
OR	Full	For children in the care of the Oregon Department of Human Services (DHS) through a voluntary placement or custody agreement, parents or legal guardians must consent to the use of psychotropic drugs. However, if the parents have signed a release agreement, then the department may consent. For children placed in legal custody of the Oregon DHS, or where the department is the legal guardian, then child welfare agency officials may consent to the use of psychotropic drugs. In any case, children 14 years or older may also consent themselves.

State	Extent	Description
TX	Full	Any individual or state department designated by name in a court order (which may include parent, relative, foster parent, or others) can give consent for psychotropic drug treatment. If the Department of Family and Protective Services (DFPS) is named, the department designates both a primary medical consenter and a back-up medical consenter (typically emergency shelter employees, live-in caregivers, relatives, or caseworkers). Children at least 16 years old may also consent themselves, if the court determines the child has the capacity to consent.
AACAP guideline		**Establish a mechanism to obtain assent for psychotropic medication management from minors when possible [minimal].[a]**
FL	Full	Since 2010, prescribers are required to determine if minor can give assent and records decision in child's medical report.
MD	Full	If a child is prescribed psychotropic medication and is development-tally able to understand the usage and effects of the medication, the child should be a part of the process and able to exercise their right to take the medication. If the child is not of age he or she can refuse medication— the assent or dissent to take medication is documented in the child's case record
MA	No	
MI	No	
OR	No	
TX	Full	DFPS policy requires all children's care with them in a development-tally appropriate way and obtain their input.
AACAP guideline		**Obtain simply written psycho-educational materials and medication information sheets to facilitate the consent process [recommended].**
FL	Full	Florida has an online guide to children's mental consent process. In addition, the child's medical consent process. The Florida Dependency Court Judges Bench-book includes a section on psychotropic drugs to help judges when reviewing cases during court hearings.
MD	Partial	The caseworker must provide information, including reason prescribed and side effects, but no standard form is used information to make informed consent decisions. One form is specific to antipsychotic medications and the other form is for all other medications. The prescriber is asked to complete the form and give it to the social worker, who can
		then ask for a member of the Massachusetts DCF Health and Medical Services Team to assist in interpreting the information and if necessary, obtain additional information from the prescriber. An information form stating the risks and benefits of medications is available to caseworkers upon request.
MA	Full	There are two documents staff can use to assist in collecting
MI	No	Although there are no psycho-educational materials and medication information sheets to facilitate the consent process, Michigan policy requires that the caseworker maintain a copy of the consent form used by the prescriber.
OR	Full	Since June 2010, the consent form allows prescribers to describe target symptoms, potential side effects, and alternative treatments. The Oregon DHS website also has a link to a medical chart that includes psychotropic drug benefits and side effects

Table 36. (Continued)

State	Extent	Description
TX	Full	Since February 2005, psycho-educational materials are available to consent-givers online through the Texas DFPS website.
AACAP guideline		**Establish training requirements for child welfare, court personnel and/or foster parents to help them become more effective advocates for children in their custody [ideal].**
FL	Partial	Florida DCF's partnership with the University and child welfare resources to foster parents and caseworkers. Guidelines are also compiled specifically for court personnel. Content related to psychotropic drugs is included in each module of the three tiers of required caseworker training. However, the names and indications for use of commonly prescribed psychotropic medications are not included as part of the required training.
MD	Partial	As part of the foster parent training, some local departments of social services have begun offering training on psychotropic drugs and the behaviors associated with taking the medication. However, there is no statewide training.
MA	Partial	Caseworkers and attorneys who represent parents and children are trained on the court process for obtaining authorization for antipsychotic medication and general information on the use and effect of psychotropic medications. However agency officials did not confirm whether each of the elements listed in AACAP's guidelines for training is included.
MI	No	Michigan has optional children health training for child welfare agency staff. There are plans to me develop training, but the particulars of the trainings had not been completed as of September 2011.
OR	Partial	Oregon required training as a one-time initiative in July 2010 for Child Welfare Supervisors that covered all of the AACAP best principle guidelines for training. The training was optional for nonsupervisory staff and a modified version of this course was provided at an annual conference for foster parents, Citizen Review Board, and other community partners. A webcast training has also been offered for foster parents and other child welfare staff and an updated version of the training is in the early development stages and will be provided as an ongoing training course once completed.
TX	Full	Since 2005, all consent-givers, except parents, must take training for informed consent and the provision of medical care which includes each of the training requirements listed in the AACAP best principle guidelines. The Minimum Standards for Residential Child Care Licensing requires that training for foster parents and other residential providers include these elements as well. DFPS has no authority to require court personnel to complete psychotropic medication training. However, DFPS is in the process of developing online training to include all of the training requirements noted in the AACAP guidelines and will be made available to children's child welfare system through an external website.

Source: GAO analysis of information collected through interviews with, and various documentation provided by, the selected states' Medicaid and foster care officials, and the AACAP's best principles guidelines.

[a] According to AACAP, consent is given by the person who has legal authority to make medical decisions, whereas assent is for the patient themselves if they are not legally able to make their own decisions.

[b] AACAP Best Principles Guidelines state this training should include the names and indications for use of commonly prescribed psychotropic medications, monitoring for medication effectiveness and side effects, and maintaining medication logs. Materials for this training should include a written "Guide to Psychotropic Medications" that includes many of the basic guidelines reviewed in the psychotropic medication training curriculum.

Table 37. State Oversight Laws and Policies Compared with AACAP's Best Principle Guidelines

State	Extent	Description
AACAP guide-line		**Establish guidelines for the use of psychotropic medications for children in state custody [minimal].**
FL	Partial	Evidence-based Medication Drug Guidelines for Children were developed by the Florida Mental Health Institute with input from physician researchers and are updated biennially. However, these guidelines are not specifically targeted towards children in state custody. Since 2008, the prior authorization review process requires a clinical review or second medical opinion by a child and adolescent psychiatrist for children less than 6 years of age prescribed an antipsychotic medication, in order to be reimbursed by Medicaid. Since 2010 prior authorization reviews are conducted for any antipsychotic lacking an FDA indication or acceptable evidence-base for safety and efficacy for children less than 18 years of age, and any high dose of antipsychotic medication.
MD	Partial	Beginning October 2011, the Maryland Medicaid Pharmacy Program (MMPP) implemented a peer- review authorization process to ensure the safe and effective use of antipsychotic medications in children. Claims for antipsychotic medications for children younger than the FDA approved age require a prior authorization based on the peer-review assessment. The MMPP's board-certified child psychiatrist oversees the peer-review project.
MA	Partial	Massachusetts guidelines are specific only to antipsychotic drugs. However, the majority of children in state custody are members of MassHealth and are subjected to the requirements and clinical management principles of the MassHealth Drug List, but these principles are not specific to foster children.
MI	Full	As of April 2010 Michigan adopted the guidelines established by Texas for the use of psychotropic medication for children in state custody.
OR	No	Since June 2010, annual reviews of psychotropic drugs must be conducted for all children under 6, or for any individual under 20 who remains in the care and custody of the state and who has more than two prescriptions for psychotropic drugs. The review must be performed by an individual other than the prescriber who is either a licensed medical professional, a qualified mental health professional with the authority to prescribe drugs, or a licensed pharmacist with the Drug Use Review Program. However, these are retrospective reviews that occur on an annual basis and do not take place at the time of prescription.

Table 37. (Continued)

State	Extent	Description
TX	Full	Since 2005, the Psychotropic Medication Utilization Parameters for Foster Children have been in place to serve as guidelines for the use of psychotropic drugs for children in foster care. For a child being prescribed a psychotropic medication, any of the following suggests the need for additional review: 1. Absence of a thorough assessment of child's 2. Five or more psychotropic medications prescribed concomitantly (side-effect medications are not included in this count) 3. Prescribing of: (a) Two or more concomitant antidepressants (if an additional one is used, may be reviewed but will be allowed if reasonable for the indications) (b) Two or more concomitant antipsychotic medications (c) Two or more concomitant stimulant medications (d) Three or more concomitant mood stabilizer medications Note: Polypharmacy is defined here as the use of two or more medications for the same indication. The prescription of a long-acting stimulant and an immediate release stimulant of the same chemical entity does not constitute concomitant prescribing and when switching psychotropic drugs, medication overlap and lowering the dose of an old drug while increasing the dose of a new drug may be utilized before discontinuing the first medication. 4. The prescribed psychotropic medication is not consistent with appropriate care for the diagnosed mental disorder or with documentted target symptoms usually associated with a therapeutic response to the medication prescribed. 5. Psychotropic polypharmacy for a given mental disorder is prescribed before utilizing psychotropic monotherapy. 6. The psychotropic medication dose exceeds usual recommended doses. 7. Psychotropic medications are prescribed for children of very young age, including children receiving the following medications with an age of: Antidepressants: Less than four years of age Antipsychotics: Less than four years of age Psychostimulants: Less than three years of age 8. Prescribing by a primary care provider who has not documented previous specialty training for a diagnosis other than the following (unless recommended by a psychiatrist consultant): Attention Deficit Hyperactive Disorder (ADHD) Uncomplicated anxiety disorders Uncomplicated depression
AACAP guide-line		**Oversight program includes an advisory committee to oversee a medication formulary and provide medication monitoring guidelines to practitioners who treat children in the child welfare system [ideal].[a]**
FL	Partials	The Florida Medicaid Drug Therapy Management Program for Behavioral Health (MDTMP for BH) was created in 2004 to improve the quality of behavioral health drug prescribing, improve patient adherence to therapy, reduce clinical risks, and lower cost while providing appropriate therapy. In 2006, an expert panel of psychiatrists developed evidence-based best practice guidelines for the use of psychotherapeutic drugs in children and adolescents.

State	Extent	Description
FL	Partial	The guidelines were published in October 2006 and are reviewed and updated biennially. Members of the panel include a combination of pediatric, adolescent, and adult psychiatrists as well as primary care physicians, pediatricians, DCF members, Agency for Health Care Administration (AHCA) staff and clinical pharmacists. However, the advisory committee does not include other mental health providers, consulting clinical pharmacists, family advocates or parents, or state child advocates. The advisory committee does not oversee a medication formulary or provide medication monitoring guidelines specifically for practitioners who treat children in the child welfare system. The Florida MDTMP for BH does provider outreach and the guidelines are also accessible online.
MD	Partial	The MMPP's board-certified child psychiatrist oversees the peer-review project for antipsychotic medications. However, there are no medication-monitoring guidelines specific to practitioners who treat children in the child welfare system.
MA	No	The Massachusetts Drug Utilization Review program's appropriate, medically necessary, and not likely to result in medication-related problems. However, Massachusetts does not have an advisory committee that oversees a medication formulary and monitoring guidelines specific to practitioners who treat children in the child welfare system.
MI	Partial	Michigan DHS established a Child Welfare Health Advisory Board in June 2010 and a subcommittee from that group meets to discuss the oversight of psychotropic medication including monitoring guidelines. Members of the subcommittee include agency and community child and adolescent psychiatrists, pediatricians, other mental health providers, and state child advocates. However, the subcommittee does not include consulting clinical pharmacists, and family advocates or parents. The group met in 2010, and it was determined that the pharmacy claims data were needed to move forward and that the group would not meet again until they were available. The advisory committee planned to meet again in October 2011 after receiving a second set of data. There is not a separate formulary for children in state custody.
OR	No	Oregon accesses the Drug Use Review (DUR) in the Division of Medical Assistance Programs. DUR is a program designed to measure and assess the proper utilization, quality, therapy, medical appropriateness, appropriate selection and cost of prescribed medication through evaluation of claims data. However, Oregon does not have an advisory committee that oversees a medication formulary and monitoring guidelines specific to practitioners who treat children in the child welfare system.
TX	Partial	In 2004, an advisory committee convened and issued a report recommending that parameters and oversight for psychotropic medications for children in foster care be put into place. In 2005 the Psychotropic Medication Utilization Parameters for Foster Children were released. The most recent update to the parameters was released in December 2010. Members of the advisory committee who update the parameters on a biennial basis as necessary include agency and community child and adolescent psychiatrists, pediatricians, other mental health providers, consulting clinical pharmacists, and family advocates or parents, but do not include state child advocates. However, according to agency officials Texas is initiating a new psychotropic medication workgroup that will include state child advocates and judges in addition to the current members. The

Table 37. (Continued)

State	Extent	Description
		Psychotropic Medication Monitoring Group, comprised of various health care professionals, reviews ongoing monitoring conducted by consulting child psychiatrists. An annual report on psychotropic medication utilization is posted online and a panel of experts reviews and updates the parameters periodically based on the most current evidence-based literature available at the time of publication.
AACAP guideline		**Oversight program monitors the rate and types of psychotropic medication usage and the rate of adverse reactions among youth in state custody [ideal].**
FL	Partial	Florida DCF has two recurring file exchanges with Florida's (AHCA). One file is used to identify and verify those children who are enrolled in the prepaid Mental health program. The second file exchange is a Psych Meds Match report that recurs monthly. This report is used to validate the recording of psychotropic medications. Florida DCF provides a list of all children who are active in in-home or out-of-home care to The third party matches against their pharmacy data and reports back all psychotropic medications prescribed for the last 3 months. This information is subsequently provided to the local agencies for monitoring. Florida DCF also provides a weekly report of all children prescribed psychotropic medications (according to the child welfare record) and a corresponding list report that includes every child by name so that regions and management can address individual cases as needed. Supervisors review cases every 30 days and may address issues at that time. The report is completed for all psychotropic medications for all children 0-17 years of age and supervisory reviews are done on all children. The Florida Mental Health Institute at the University of South Florida performs retrospective prescription claims reviews for AHCA to determine the rate and types of psychotropic drugs used for Medicaid eligible children in the child welfare system. However, Florida DCF does not monitor the rate and types of psychotropic medication in relation to the state guidelines and does not monitor and review adverse reactions at the aggregate level.
MD	Partial	According to an agency official, data on rate and types of psychotropic medication usage are gathered for all children in the child welfare system in a collaborative effort between the Departments of Human Resources (Child Welfare) and Health and Mental Hygiene, and the University of Maryland Schools of Pharmacy, Social Work and Medicine. However, there is not a uniform system in place among local departments of social services to monitor the rate of adverse reactions.
MA	Partial	Unstable and medically complex children receive home visits from a pediatric nurse practitioner. Also, when a court authorizes antipsychotic medication, it appoints a Guardian ad Litem to monitor the use of the medication and it sets periodic— usually every 6 months— reviews of the usage and impact of the medication, including any adverse reactions.
MI	Partial	Michigan DHS completed an interagency agreement for data sharing with the Michigan Department of Community Health (DCH) to review foster children's However, Michigan DHS was unable to build reliable reports with the first data set received April 2011 and there is no process to monitor and review adverse reactions.

State	Extent	Description
OR	Partial	As of June 2010, an annual review of psychotropic medications by an individual other than the prescriber is performed when: (a) a child or young adult has more than two prescriptions for psychotropic medications; or (b) a child is under 6 years of age. The annual review guidelines have been used as a threshold for review or additional review on an individual basis. There is no macro level review of foster trends across the entire foster care population and no aggregate reviews of adverse reactions to medications. Prior to 2010 the department enacted a number of different informal strategies to better understand and inform the process which concluded with the development of the rules now in place.
TX	Partial	In June 2006, a report on the use of psychotropic medications in Texas foster children was released. This macro level analysis reports the rate and types of various psychotropic prescribing practices and is updated and reported on an annual basis. However, adverse reactions are not tracked and reviewed on a macro level.
AACAP guideline		**Oversight program establishes a process to review non-standard, unusual, and/or experimental psychiatric interventions with children who are in state custody [ideal].**
FL	Partial	A preconsent review by a consultant child psychiatrist is obtained prior to the prescription of a psychotropic medication for any child under 11 years of age who is prescribed two or more psychotropic medications and who is in the custody of the department in out-of-home care. The results of the review by the consultant child psychiatrist are provided to the child and to the person who has legal authority to provide express and informed consent or the judge who is providing the court order for treatment with a psychotropic medication. Florida DCF may utilize the - consent review contract with the University of Florida or may contract locally with a child psychiatrist. The University of Florida has at least two certified child psychiatrists on staff who review the medications identified by Florida DCF for additional review. The child psychiatrists can contact the prescriber and request more information or recommend alternative treatment options as necessary. However, the prescribing physician is permitted by law to fill the prescription using their own discretion regardless of the child psychiatrists' recommendation.
MD	Partial	A child and adolescent psychiatrist who is on the faculty at Johns Hopkins University School of Medicine monitors all psychotropic medication use for children entering foster care in Baltimore City. However, this practice is not statewide.
MA	Partial	For extraordinary, complex, risky, or novel treatment, Massachusetts DCF is required to get the consent of the parents (if the child is in the department's the department's custody). However, the only meet these criteria is antipsychotic medications.
MI	Full	The Michigan DHS oversight program flags pharmacy claims when the prescribing of psychotropic medication falls outside of established guide-lines. Current reviews are conducted on prescribing practices including: four or more psychotropic medications prescribed concomitantly; prescribing two or more concomitant antidepressant medications, two or more concomitant antipsychotic medications, two or more concomitant stimulant medications, or two or more concomitant mood stabilizer medi-cations; psychotropic medication dose exceeds usually recommended dose; and psychotropic medications prescribed for children 5 years and

Table 37. (Continued)

State	Extent	Description
		under. In addition, Michigan DHS hired 25 health liaison officers to serve as health care advocates for foster children and help assist in the review and oversight process of psychotropic medications under the direction of the Michigan DHS medical consultant.
OR	Partial	Oregon's annual review guidelines have been used as a threshold for review or additional review on an individual basis.
TX	Full	Since April 2008, State of Texas Access Reform (STAR) Health Service Managers perform health assessments on foster children to identify those who have medication regimens which appear to be outside the Psychotropic Medication Utilization Parameters.
AACAP guideline		**Oversight program collects and analyzes data and makes quarterly reports to the state or county child welfare agency regarding the rates and types of psychotropic medication use. These data are made available to clinicians in the state to improve the quality of care provided [ideal].**
FL	Partial	Florida DCF reports the number of children on psychotropic medications, the number of children who received informed consent, and the demographics of those cases on a weekly basis to management. Florida DCF monitors the number of children prescribed psychotropic medications and whether valid express and informed consent were obtained or court authorized, but does not monitor and report the rates and types of psychotropic medications prescribed. The state conducts quarterly quality assurance reviews of all community-based care agencies. Cases are randomly selected for a comprehensive quality assurance review and if the child is on psychotropic medications, the reviewer is required to determine if the case management organization complied with statute and Florida Administrative Code. All quality assurance reports are accessible online. Florida DCF also publishes an annual report of findings.
MD	Partial	The oversight program used in Baltimore City collects and analyzes data and makes reports to the state and the Baltimore City Child Welfare Department. However, this practice is not statewide.
MA	Partial	Individual cases are reviewed quarterly, but macro-level reports are not done regularly. However, episodic reports have been issued on the rates and types of psychotropic medication for specific drug types and age ranges that include foster children.
MI	No	There is a plan to look at the claims data systemically, but it has not yet been determined how the reports will be developed or shared. Those decisions will be made by the Child Welfare Health Advisory Board's subcommittee.
OR	No	Medication logs are reviewed monthly on an individual basis by the caseworker, but no macro-level report is available to improve the quality of care.
TX	Full	Quarterly reports are reviewed by the Psychotropic Medication Monitoring Group, which is chaired by DFPS. These reports include the percentile of children in foster care on psychotropic medications and the percentile that are outside parameters (receiving any psychotropic medications under age 4 years, two of more of the same class and/or five or more of the same class). Annually, at the end of each state fiscal year, a report specific to foster children is generated from Medicaid prescription data and posted on the Texas Health and Human Services Commission website for use by clinicians and other stakeholders.

State	Extent	Description
AACAP guideline		**Maintain an ongoing record of diagnoses, height and weight, allergies, medical history, ongoing medical problem list, psychotropic medications, and adverse medication reactions that are easily available to treating clinicians 24 hours a day [ideal].**
FL	Partial	Florida maintains a resource record as the child's available and accessible medical and psychological information— including behavioral health information— pertaining to the child. The resource record is a hard copy form maintained in the foster home. However, the states Automated Child Welfare Information System includes medical information and most child welfare agencies store documents electronically to maintain copies of medical records. The electronic systems that store critical information such as immunizations and medical history are accessible 24 hours a day. However, record of diagnosis, height and weight, allergies, medical history, ongoing medical problem list, psychotropic medications, and adverse medication reactions are specifically required to be maintained.
MD	Full	Each child that enters out-of-home placement is given a medical passport. This passport serves as a record of the child's previous and current resource (e.g., foster parents or group home) and is carried to every medical appointment to be reviewed if necessary by the health care provider. Each medical visit, medication, and immunization is documented in the passport along with diagnoses, height and weight, allergies, medical history, ongoing medical problem list, psychotropic medications, and adverse medication reactions. An additional copy of the passport is kept in the child's case record maintained at the child's placement it is available it is available 24 hours a day for emergencies.
MA	Partial	Massachusetts DCF requires the use of a "medical passport" for all children in substitute care. The medical passport records pertinent and available medical/dental/mental health and developmental data about the child. Department social workers and medical providers complete relevant portions of the passport. The passports are held by the substitute care provider and remain with the child for the duration of his or her placement. If a child moves to a new substitute care placement or returns home, the medical passport moves with the child. However, the medical passport does not include height and weight, adverse reactions, or an ongoing medical problem list.
MI	Full	Each foster child is provided a medical passport that records all of the elements recommended by AACAP. The passport is a paper document and is provided to the foster parents to ensure health information is updated as necessary. The passport stays with the child over time, but it is the responsibility of the foster parents to make sure the passport stays updated and is made available to treating clinicians.
OR	Partial	Oregon has medical information and a health care record for the child in foster care. However, these records may not be inclusive of all the child's — which may be with other medical offices— and they are not accessible 24 hours a day to health care providers.
TX	Partial	As of April 2008, a web-based electronic health record system maintains health information for foster children and is available to treating clinicians 24 hours a day. The electronic health record system records an ongoing record of diagnoses, medical history, and psychotropic medications, but the adverse medication reactions, height and weight, and allergies are optional and not all health care providers enter this information. An ongoing medical problem list is not recorded in the electronic health record system.

Source: GAO analysis of information collected through interviews with, and various documentation provided by, the selected states' Medicaid and foster care officials, and the AACAP's best principles guidelines.

[a] AACAP describes advisory committees as composed of agency and community child and adolescent psychiatrists, pediatricians, other mental health providers, consulting clinical pharmacists, family advocates or parents, and state child advocates.

Table 38. State Consultation Programs Compared with AACAP's Best Principle Guidelines

State	Extent	Description
AACAP guideline		**Design a consultation program administered by child and adolescent psychiatrists. This program provides consultation by child and adolescent psychiatrists to the persons or agency that is responsible for consenting for treatment with psychotropic medications [recommended].[a]**
FL	Full	Starting in 2004, the MedConsult line was made available for families, guardians, and the courts to consult with board-certified child psychiatrists via telephone. The purpose of the MedConsult line is to assist decision makers who give express and informed consent for psychotropic medication for dependent children or children enrolled in the Behavioral Health Network. The MedConsult Line is available Monday through Friday 9:00 am until 5:00 pm. The court may order
		additional medical consultation, including consultation with the MedConsult line at the University of Florida, if available, or require the department to obtain a second opinion within a reasonable timeframe as established by the court, not to exceed 21 calendar days, after such order based upon consideration of the best interests of the child. The MedConsult line is not a second opinion and participation is voluntary. The kind of information provided include indicated uses, usual and customary practices, dose ranges, starting dose, FDA Box Warnings, on-or off-label use, any precautions such as EKGs, and lab work.
MD	No	
MA	Partial	The Massachusetts Department of Mental Health (DMH) has six child psychiatrists who are available to provide consultations on a part-time basis. In addition, Massachusetts DCF has a part-time child psychiatrist on staff who is available for consultation on individual cases and provides consultation to the agency senior managers. Pharmacists are also available to consult with consent-giver s if the child is enrolled on MassHealth. A pharmacist is available via phone to provide information regarding the drug history, provide an opinion on proposed medications— including interactions between multiple medications— make consent recommendations, and/or call the prescriber to ask questions and seek additional information.
OR	Partial	As of February 2009, child welfare agency officials give consent for children placed in legal custody of Oregon DHS, or where the department is the legal guardian, and have access to a consulting child and adolescent psychiatrist on a part-time basis.

State	Extent	Description
TX	Partial	The DFPS Medical Director who is a board-certified child and adolescent psychiatrist, consults with CPS staff regarding policy, procedures, training materials and complex cases. Under the guidance of the DFPS Medical Director, the CPS Division Administrator for Medical Services and the Regional Nurse Consultants also provide guidance and education to staff that consent to a psychotropic medications and consult on specific cases when necessary or when requested.
AACAP guideline		**The consultation program provides consultations by child and adolescent psychiatrists to, and at the request of, physicians treating this difficult patient population [recommended].**
FL	Full	The MedConsult line is available to physicians who seek consultations by child and adolescent psychiatrists.
MD	Partial	A child and adolescent psychiatrist consults with prescribers for youth entering Baltimore City Child Welfare. MMPP has contracted with the University of Maryland (UMD) Division of Child and Adolescent Psychiatry and School of Pharmacy to provide call center services. UMD utilizes psychiatrists and pharmacists to answer calls from Medicaid prescribers who prescribe antipsychotic medications off-label to children and provide reviews of patient profiles to determine if the program will approve or deny the claim. However, these reviews are only for antipsychotic drugs and do not include other psychotropic drugs.
MA	Full	As of December 2005, the Massachusetts Child Psychiatry Access Project (MCPAP) was put in place, which allows pediatricians to have access to consultations with child and adolescent psychiatrists by phone on weekdays between 9 a.m. and 5 p.m., within 30 minutes of the request.
MI	No	
OR	No	The Oregon Psychiatric Access Line for Kids project is under development which would allow primary care physicians and nurse practitioners to consult with child psychiatrists as needed. Agency officials told us that future implementation is dependent on finding a long-term funding source. Neither the Oregon Foster children program nor the state Medicaid agency currently uses this program.
TX	No	Child psychiatrists with Texas STAR health consult with prescribing physicians as part of the psychotropic medication utilization review process. However, these consultations are not conducted at the request of treating physicians as recommended by AACAP.
AACAP guideline		**The consultation program conducts face-to-face evaluations of youth by child and adolescent psychiatrists at the request of the child welfare agency, the juvenile court, or other state or county agencies empowered by law to consent for treatment with psychotropic medications when concerns have been raised about the pharmacological regimen [recommended].**
FL, MD	No	
MA	Full	Massachusetts DCF mental health specialists are able to arrange consultations or evaluations if needed and the Juvenile Courts have access to Juvenile Court Clinics where evaluations can be conducted.
MI, OR	No	
TX	Full	Since April 2008, the psychotropic medication utilization review process is triggered when a medication regimens are outside the parameters or when certain criteria are met, including at the request of CPS nurse consultants, caseworkers, court appointed special advocates, foster parents, attorneys, residential child care providers, and at the request of the court.

Source: GAO analysis of information collected through interviews with, and various documentation provided by, the selected states' Medicaid and foster care officials, and the AACAP's best principles guidelines.

[a] Massachusetts, Oregon, and Texas received a partial categorization because the consultation programs do not ensure all possible consent-givers have access to consultations with a child and adolescent psychiatrist. For example, when parent(s) have retained their rights to consent for their child's medication and the child enters foster care through a voluntary placement agreement. In addition, consultations in Massachusetts and Oregon are only available to agency officials on a part- time basis.

Table 39. State Information-Sharing Laws and Policies Compared with AACAP's Best Principle Guidelines

State	Extent	Description
AACAP guideline		**Create a website to provide ready access for clinicians, foster parents, and other caregivers to pertinent policies and procedures governing psychotropic medication management [ideal].**
FL	Full	Florida DCF has partnered with the University of South Florida to implement Advancement of Child Welfare Practice to provide needed information and support to professional child welfare stakeholders. The website includes policies and procedures regulating psychotropic drug management.
MD	No	
MA	Full	The official website of the Executive Office of Health and Human Services (EOHHS) includes policies and procedures governing psychotropic medication management.
MI	No	
OR	Full	Oregon developed a website as a communication tool during the implementation of the 2010 administrative rules, but the website is not an ongoing resource for information. The website currently has information on state policies and procedures governing the use of psychotropic drugs.
TX	Full	As of September 2005, DFPS posted the Psychotropic Medication Utilization Parameters for Foster Children on the agency's website. Also, DFPS underlying the parameters into each residential child-care contract. The residential contract is revised each year and posted on the website.
AACAP guideline		**Website includes psycho-educational materials [ideal].**
FL	Full	Florida's Center for the Advancement of Child educational materials about psychotropic drugs.
MD	No	
MA	Full	The official website of EOHHS includes web links to psycho-educational materials and publications.
MI	No	According to an agency official, Michigan DHS added a Health Information and Resource page to its internal website that Michigan DHS staff can access. The

State	Extent	Description
		website is updated by the Health, Education, and Youth Unit and was activated in January 2011. However, this information is not available to external caregivers such as clinicians.[a]
OR	Full	Oregon's hat can be used as a psychotropic medication website links to medication reference tool.
TX	Full	As of February of 2005, DFPS posted the Psychotropic Medication Utilization Parameters for Foster Children on their website. The parameters describe appropriate practice for prescribers and literature references. Since the Summer of 2007, DFPS has posted tables addressing medication uses, dosages and possible side effects on the agency website.
AACAP guideline		**Website includes consent forms [ideal].**
FL	Full	Florida's Center for the Advancement of Child Welfare Practice website includes a consent form.
MD	No	
MA	No	
MI	No	
OR	Full	Oregon's official website includes a consent
TX	No	DFPS does not have a standardized form that all prescribing health care providers are required to use. Each health care provider documents consent in his or her office-based medical record.
AACAP guideline		**Website includes adverse effect rating forms [ideal].**
FL	No	
MD	No	
MA	No	
MI	No	
OR	No	
TX	No	
AACAP guideline		**Website includes reports on prescription patterns for psychotropic medications [ideal].**
FL	No	Although Florida's Center for the Advancement prescribing patterns, Florida's patterns and tracks informed consent DCF website as of 2009.
MD	No	
MA	No	
MI	No	
OR	No	
TX	Full	Annual outcomes regarding prescribing patterns are posted on the website.
AACAP Guideline		**Website includes links to helpful, accurate, and ethical websites about child and adolescent psychi-atric diagnoses and psychotropic medications [ideal].**
FL	Full	The website includes links to other informative publications and news stories related to foster children and psychotropic medications.
MD	No	
MA	No	

Table 38. (Continued)

State	Extent	Description
MI	No	Agency officials said that Michigan DHS has a draft policy to link publications from the National Institute of Mental Health to the Michigan DHS website to give workers up-to-date information about child and adolescent psychiatric diagnoses and psychotropic medications.
OR	No	
TX	Full	The website includes links to state and national sites that have information on medication guidelines and diagnoses of psychotropic medications.

Source: GAO analysis of information collected through interviews with, and various documentation provided by, the selected states' Medicaid and foster care officials, and the AACAP's best principles guidelines.

[a] This information was provided by Michigan state officials and was not tested to ensure effective implementation.

End Notes

[1] GAO, *Foster Care: State Practices for Assessing Health Needs, Facilitating Service Delivery, and Monitoring*, GAO-09-26 (Washington, D.C.: Feb. 6, 2009).

[2] Medicaid programs vary from state to state.

[3] National Institute of Mental Health, *Treatment of Children with Mental Illness, NIH Publication No. 09-4702* (Bethesda, Md.: Revised 2009).

[4] For example, see Medicaid Medical Directors Learning Network and Rutgers Center for Education and Research on Mental Health Therapeutics, *Antipsychotic Medication Use in Medicaid Children and Adolescents: Report and Resource Guide from a 16-State Study* MMDLN/Rutgers CERTs, Publication 1 (July 2010).

[5] AACAP guidelines are available at http://www.aacap.org/galleries/PracticeInformation/Foster Care_ BestPrinciples_FINAL.pdf

[6] Pub. L. No. 112-34, § 101(b)(2), 125 Stat. 369.

[7] Some states' prescription drugs are covered by Medicaid managed care plans in which drug payments are included in the capitated payments that plans receive from states. For this review, we selected states that cover psychotropic medications largely under fee-for-service programs so that individual drug claims could be analyzed. In Michigan, Oregon, and Texas, psychotropic medications were primarily paid on a fee-for-service basis. In Florida and Massachusetts, psychotropic prescription claims for most foster children were paid on a fee-for-service basis, with the remaining children largely covered by managed care. In Florida, about 60 percent of foster children and 45 percent of nonfoster children had their prescriptions covered only on a fee-for-service basis during 2008. In Massachusetts, the percentages were about 72 percent for foster children and about 42 percent for nonfoster children. For these two states, our analysis is not applicable to the entire state's foster care or fee-for-service data, we were more likely to identify psychotropic prescriptions for foster children during calendar year 2008 than for nonfoster children. Appendix IV shows how rates of psychotropic prescriptions are affected by the length of time a child is covered under a Medicaid fee-for-service program.

[8] According to our experts, these medications, such as anticonvulsants, are likely being prescribed to treat mental health conditions when combined with another psychotropic medication.

[9] GAO, *Foster Care: State Practices for Assessing Health Needs, Facilitating Service Delivery, and Monitoring Children's Care*, GAO-09-26 (Washington, D.C.: Feb. 6, 2009).

[10] We also examined Maryland, but found that its 2008 data on foster children were not sufficiently reliable for this study. State officials told us that Maryland's transition to a new records system in 2007 resulted in incorrect and missing data for foster children. A state audit in 2008 reported duplicate records with different identifying numbers for the same child, records showing children who had exited foster care as still enrolled in the program, and personal information for the mother recorded as that of the child. Our analysis of the data Maryland provided to us identified 8,869 children in foster care as of September 30, 2008—about 16 percent more than the 7,613 children that Maryland reported to ACF that year. However, audit reports for Maryland indicated that the state had taken some corrective actions as of March 2011.

[11] Based on our analysis of Medicaid fee-for-service claims data, these five states spent over $317 million on psychotropic drugs for nonfoster children and about $59 million on psychotropic drugs for foster children (in care 30 days or more) during 2008. This amount paid includes only claims paid for by a fee-for-service program and does not include manufacturer rebates or costs such as managed care (e.g., health maintenance organization (HMO)).

[12] For example, see Leslie et al, *Multi-State Study on Psychotropic Medication Oversight in Foster Care*, Tufts Clinical and Translational Science Institute (Boston, Mass: 2010).

[13] According to our experts, medications are approved based on therapeutic research and doses above the recommended level have generally not been shown to be safe or effective.

[14] The kinds of drugs included in prescription data reported to CMS in 2008 varied by state. Because the claims data we obtained from CMS contained fewer types of medications for Michigan and Oregon, we may understate the rates of psychotropic prescriptions for both foster and nonfoster children in those states. While rates of psychotropic prescriptions are not comparable across states, they are comparable between foster and nonfoster children within the same state. Similarly, the ratios of prescriptions to foster children to prescriptions to nonfoster children are comparable across states.

[15] In Florida, nonfoster children were in fee-for-service Medicaid an average of 2 months less than foster children. Therefore, the number of nonfoster children with psychotropic prescriptions may be understated.

[16] S. dosReis et al., *Mental Health Services for Youths in Foster Care and Disabled Youths*, Am J Public Health, 2001, 91(7): pp 1094-9.

[17] Children in states that required CPS to initially contact the family before the study's field staff were excluded from the study. Those states are not represented. See National Survey of Child and Adolescent Well-Being (NSCAW), No. 7: *Special Health Care Needs Among Children in Child Welfare*, Office of Planning, Research and Evaluation, Administration for Children and Families (Washington, D.C.: 2007).

[18] Children in states that required CPS to initially contact the family before the study's field staff were excluded from the study. Those states are not represented. See B.J. Burns et al., *Mental Health Need and Access to Mental Health Services by Youths Involved with Child Welfare: A National Survey*, Journal of the American Academy of Child and Adolescent Psychiatry, 43 (2004), pp. 960-70.

[19] As we have previously reported, some steps have been taken to address the lack of drug research in the pediatric population. For example, as part of the Food and Drug Administration Amendments Act of 2007, Congress reauthorized two laws, the Pediatric Research Equity Act (PREA) and the Best Pharmaceuticals for Children Act (BPCA). The PREA requires that sponsors conduct pediatric studies for certain products unless the FDA grants a waiver or deferral. *See GAO, Pediatric Research: Products Studied under Two Related Laws, but Improved Tracking Needed by FDA*, GAO-1 1-457 (Washington, D.C.: May 2011).

[20] GAO, *Foster Care: State Practices for Assessing Health Needs, Facilitating Service Delivery, and Monitoring Children's Care*, GAO-09-26 (Washington, D.C.: Feb. 6, 2009).

[21] For example, see Leslie et al., *Multi-State Study on Psychotropic Medication Oversight in Foster Care*, Tufts Clinical and Translational Science Institute (Boston, Mass.: 2010).

[22] Leslie et al, *Multi-State Study on Psychotropic Medication Oversight in Foster Care*, Tufts Clinical and Translational Science Institute (Boston, Mass.: 2010).

[23] According to one of our experts, this may be justified in rare cases of children with serious, complex mental health issues.

[24] These indicators are similar to those used by Texas to identify cases for further review, and were cited by our experts as indicators of potential health risks.

[25] In our analysis of rates of psychotropic prescriptions, we included stimulants (e.g., ADHD drugs), anti-anxiety drugs, antidepressants, antipsychotics, hypnotics, mood stabilizers, and medications containing combinations of these drug classes. Other psychotropic drugs, such as anticonvulsants and alpha agonists, may be used to treat both physical and mental health conditions. However, because they are more likely to be used for mental health indications when combined with another psychotropic drug, we included them in our concomitant analyses when combined with a second psychotropic drug. See app. I for more details explaining how the concomitant analysis was conducted to eliminate cases in which a patient began taking a new drug without finishing the previous supply, thereby creating the appearance of concurrent use.

[26] For example, see Zito et al., *Psychotropic Medication Patterns Among Youth in Foster Care*, Pediatrics 2008; Volume 121; pp.157-163.

[27] For this analysis, we used dosage guidelines developed by the state of Texas based on FDA-approved drug labels, where available, for 33 drugs. For additional information, see Heiligenstein, *Psychotropic Medication Utilization Parameters for Foster Children*, Office of the Commissioner, Texas Department of Family and Protective Services (Austin, Tex.: December 2010).

[28] According to one of our experts, the effect of psychotropic medications has not been proven to be safe or effective above the maximum recommended dose by an FDA review. At lower dosages, psychotropic medications generally show an increase in efficacy with an increase in dose, but this dose-response relationship changes as the dose increases. At higher dosages, increasing doses of medications are often accompanied by an increased risk in adverse effects with little or no added benefit.

[29] While the data we used for this analysis were generally reliable, the date-of-birth field was blank for some records. The number of foster infants, in particular, captured in the claims data may be underreported. It is also possible that a small number of Medicaid and foster care records may contain inaccurate personal data or prescription information likely resulting from data entry errors. See app. I on our assessment of data reliability.

[30] Experts also noted that some of these prescriptions may have been written with the intention of treating an uninsured parent or sibling. It is not possible to determine from the data whether this was the case.

[31] Infrequent gaps may also be caused by a serious illness that prevents the patient from taking the medication as prescribed, or patients who choose to discontinue a medication because of side effects.

[32] G. Chouinard, *Issues in the clinical use of benzodiazepines: potency, withdrawal, and rebound*, J Clin Psychiatry, 2004; 65 Suppl 5: pp. 7-12.

[33] SSRIs are antidepressants.

[34] S. Hosenbocus and R. *Chahal, SSRIs and SNRIs: A review of the Discontinuation Syndrome in Children and Adolescents*, J Can Acad Child Adolesc Psychiatry (February 2011) 20(1): pp. 60-67.

[35] National Institute of Mental Health, *Mental Health Medications*, U.S. Department of Health and Human Services (Bethesda, Md.: Revised 2008).

[36] Child and Family Services Improvement and Innovation Act, Pub. L. No. 112-34, § 101(b)(2), 125 Stat. 369 (2011).

[37] CFSRs, which occur on a regular and recurring basis in every state (generally every 2 to 5 years depending on the results of the prior review), are the central and most comprehensive component of federal efforts to determine state compliance with federal child welfare requirements. ACF also reviews states' progress related to areas found not to be in substantial conformity with federal requirements based on the last CFSR, generally on an annual basis.

[38] In order to be eligible for certain federal child welfare grants, state child welfare agencies are required to develop a plan for ongoing oversight and coordination of health care services for foster children, including mental health, in coordination with the state Medicaid agency, pediatricians, other health care experts, and child welfare experts. See 42 U.S.C. § 622(b)(15). Among other things, the state plans must also include the oversight of prescription drugs, and how the agency actively consults and involves physicians and other professionals in assessing the health and well-being of children in foster care in determining appropriate medical treatment for the children.

[39] Each of the six states reviewed performs a drug utilization review during the prescription claims process to promote patient safety, reduce costs, and prevent fraud and abuse as required by the Omnibus Budget Reconciliation Act (OBRA) of 1990 (Pub. L. No. 101-508, § 4401, 104 Stat. 1388, § 1388-143. (1990)). States were encouraged by enhanced federal funding to design and install point-of-sale electronic claims management systems that interface with their Medicaid Management Information Systems (MMIS) operations. The annual report requirement is used to assess patient safety, provider prescribing habits, and dollars saved by avoidance of problems such as drug-drug interactions, drug-disease interactions, therapeutic duplication, and overprescribing by providers. However, the extent to which a state's DUR process included reviews of psychotropic drugs varied across our states and the DUR process is not focused on the foster child population specifically.

[40] M.W. Naylor, et al., *Psychotropic Medication Management for Youth in State Care: Consent, Oversight, and Policy Considerations*, Child Welfare V 86, 5 (2007) pp.175-1 92.

[41] Primary care provider prescriptions were not flagged when treating ADHD, uncomplicated depression, and uncomplicated anxiety disorders.

[42] Beginning October 2011, the Maryland Medicaid Pharmacy Program (MMPP) implemented a peer-review authorization process to ensure the safe and effective use of antipsychotic medications in children. Claims for antipsychotic medications that are for children younger than the FDA-approved age require prior authorization (PA) based on the peer-review assessment. The MMPP's board-certified child psychiatrist oversees the peer-review project. According to a state agency official, a child and adolescent psychiatrist who is faculty at Johns Hopkins University School of Medicine monitors all psychotropic medication use for children entering foster care in Baltimore City. However, this practice is not statewide.

[43] According to the Center's website, its mission is to support and facilitate the identification, expansion, and transfer of expert knowledge and best practices in child welfare case practice, direct services, management, finances, policy, and organizational development to child welfare and child protection stakeholders throughout Florida.

[44] However, we determined through data tests, interviews, and reviews of state audit reports that data on children in Maryland foster care during 2008 were unreliable. Maryland data were not included in the data analysis portion of this report.

[45] States with fee-for-service carve outs for psychotropic medications pay providers directly for these medications, and manage the resulting claims in a centralized data set. States without prescription carve outs used managed care organizations to oversee and pay for prescriptions, resulting in numerous, noncentralized data sets that would have inhibited our ability to identify psychotropic drugs for this analysis.

[46] Approved drugs lists were either the state's formulary or preferred drug list.

[47] Although some medications may be prescribed on an "as needed" basis, these types of prescriptions are not distinguished in the data. In our analysis of doses exceeding levels recommended by the FDA and medical literature, we count all medications as though they were taken on a daily basis.

[48] According to one of our experts, these secondary medications are likely used to treat physical symptoms when prescribed alone, but when paired with another psychotropic medication, they are likely used for mental health.

[49] In Florida, about 60 percent of foster children and 45 percent of nonfoster children had their prescriptions covered only on a fee-for-service basis during 2008. In Massachusetts, the percentages were about 72 percent for foster children and about 42 percent for nonfoster children. For these two states, our analysis is not applicable to the entire state's foster care or Medicaid program.

[50] Thomson Reuters' Red BookTM is a medical resource for healthcare professionals for current information on medications.

[51] Calculating the number of prescriptions on a monthly rather than daily basis may result in an underestimate of concomitant prescriptions for individuals with continuous prescriptions that did not cover 84 days during 3 calendar months.

[52] For a comprehensive list of mental health medication categories, uses, and side effects, see National Institute of Mental Health, Mental Health Medications, U.S. Department of Health and Human Services (Bethesda, Md.: Revised 2008).

[53] For our analysis of concomitant use, we also included several drugs from the following categories: certain anti-anxiety drugs, anticonvulsants, anti-enuretics, antiparkinson drugs, and sleep aids.

[54] Combination drugs have two different classes of drugs in a single dose. For example, Symbyax contains olanzepine and fluoxetine, an antipsychotic and an antidepressant. This medication is used to treat depression with bipolar I disorder or depression that does not respond to other medicines. These drugs have side effects similar to their component medications.

[55] Some benzodiazepines may be prescribed for insomnia, and therefore may also be considered hypnotics.

[56] Some medications developed to treat depression, such as selective serotonin reuptake inhibitors and tricyclic antidepressants may also be used to treat anxiety disorders.

[57] Some anti-anxiety medications may also be considered hypnotics. For example, in this report we categorize clonazepam (Klonopin), lorazepam (Ativan), and alprazolam (Xanax) as anti-anxiety medications, but they may also be used for insomnia.

[58] For example, Symbyax contains olanzapine and fluoxetine, an antipsychotic and an antidepressant, in a single dose.

In: Medicating Foster Care Children... ISBN: 978-1- 61942-889-8
Editors: R. L. Ray and M. A. Watkins

Chapter 2

MEDICATING FOSTER CHILDREN HEARING-BROWN STATEMENT*

Scott Brown

"The Financial and Societal Costs of Medicating America's Foster Children"

December 1, 2011

Senator Carper, thank you for holding this important hearing today.

Foster children, often being removed from neglectful or abusive homes, are one of the country's most vulnerable populations. With the often traumatic circumstances that define their early lives, it is no wonder studies show their tendency for more mental health conditions than other children. Facing these and other significant challenges surrounding foster care programs, state authorities, caseworkers, and parents, are given few options on appropriate treatments. As our witnesses will discuss today, these options often include prescribing heavy-duty psychotropic drugs such as antidepressants and, in some cases, even antipsychotics – drugs which have little research available supporting their use in children.

---

* This is an edited, reformatted and augmented version of the statement of Senator Scott Brown, Ranking Member, before the Committee on Homeland Security and Governmental Affairs, Hearing on "The Financial and Societal Costs of Medicating America's Foster Children."

While the use of psychotropic medications has been shown to effectively treat mental disorders, the side-effects and risks they pose, specifically to children, are not well understood. This is why we asked GAO to look into this issue more closely and their investigation has produced some alarming results. Not only are foster children being prescribed psychotropic drugs at a higher rate than non-foster kids in general, but also in ways that hold significantly higher risks, such as multiple medications at once or in amounts exceeding FDA recommendations. In Massachusetts, nearly 40% of the foster children population analyzed in the report was prescribed at least one psychotropic drug -- a rate almost four times that of non-foster children. In over 900 cases in Massachusetts, foster children were being prescribed three or more drugs at once. While the scope of the report does not address the appropriateness of these prescriptions on a case-by-case basis, it does reignite the debate over whether the rates of prescribing match the scientific evidence behind these medical conditions.

Regrettably, the concerns raised in the report are not just limited to foster children. Though high-risk prescribing practices for foster children were found at higher rates than non-foster children in most cases, the significantly larger population of non-foster children covered by Medicaid makes these statistics just as alarming. For instance, thousands of prescriptions -- a total of 5,265 according to the report -- were filled for infants under one year old. This is just the data from five states! In Massachusetts 49 infants were found to have been prescribed psychotropics, in some cases even antipsychotics. Though 49 is a small number compared to the total, one child infant found on these drugs should invite serious scrutiny considering that experts have found NO mental health indications for the use of psychotropic drugs in infants. As our witnesses will testify today, providing these powerful drugs to infants could result in serious adverse effects and the potential risks are simply too great.

Medicaid, which is run by states and administered by the Department of Health and Human Services, provides prescription drug coverage to foster children. As of today, HHS has limited authority to adequately oversee state monitoring programs for youths in state custody. As a result, states' comprehensive oversight policies are a mishmash of programs in various stages of maturity. Although HHS provides informational resources such as "best practices" to help inform state monitoring programs for children in state custody, each state is responsible for designing and implementing its own program. As GAO has examined with the five states it reviewed, many times these programs fall short of providing the comprehensive oversight that is desperately needed.

It is obvious that consistent and comprehensive guidelines in this area are necessary to more effectively treat and reduce harmful risks to children in the Medicaid program, and particularly foster children. In addition, better oversight in this area can have a broader impact in reducing fraud, waste, and abuse in Medicaid in general. I encourage HHS to rapidly endorse guidance on best practices and use its current authority to push state Medicaid and child welfare agencies to improve these programs as quickly as possible. The government has been charged to protect these children and it is not acceptable to fail them any further.

I thank the witnesses for their attendance today and look forward to a helpful discussion on how we can prevent just that. Thank you Mr. Chairman.

In: Medicating Foster Care Children...
Editors: R. L. Ray and M. A. Watkins
ISBN: 978-1- 61942-889-8

Chapter 3

MEDICATING FOSTER CHILDREN HEARING-SAMUELS TESTIMONY*

Bryan Samuels

Chairman Carper, Ranking Member Brown, and members of the subcommittee, thank you for the opportunity to testify before you this morning about the use of psychotropic medications among children in foster care. First, I would like to acknowledge the leadership demonstrated by Congress in this area already, most recently in the reauthorization of title IV-B of the Social Security Act. In September, Congress acted on an administration proposal to provide HHS with additional authority in the Child and Family Services Improvement and Innovations Act of 2011 (Public Law 112-34) to require states to address the trauma needs of children and to develop protocols for monitoring the use of psychotropic drugs among children in foster care. Other notable Congressional work includes the passage of the Fostering Connections to Success and Increasing Adoptions Act, which requires the use of medical homes and oversight of prescription medications for children in foster care, and the recent work of the Senate Caucus on Foster Youth, led by senators Landrieu and Grassley, to highlight the issue of psychotropics. In 2009, the Subcommittee on Income Security and Family Support of the House

* This is an edited, reformatted and augmented version of the statement of Bryan Sammuels, Commissioner, Administration on Children, Youth and Families, U.S. Department of Health and Human Services, before the Committee on Homeland Security and Governmental Affairs, Hearing on "The Financial and Societal Costs of Medicating America's Foster Children."

Committee on Ways and Means held a hearing on prescription psychotropic drug use among children in foster care. Additionally, I would like to thank this Committee for requesting that the Government Accountability Office review the use of psychotropics with children in foster care, as it has produced a comprehensive and useful report that can help guide ongoing action. As I have noted, much work has occurred already, and the hearing today furthers this critical conversation. Together, this work will advance the child welfare and mental health fields and truly benefit some of the most vulnerable children in our society.

During my testimony, I will address critical issues related to the use of psychotropic medication among children in foster care and outline the activities that the Department of Health and Human Services (HHS) has undertaken to improve oversight and monitoring. It is impossible to discuss the use of psychotropics without addressing the impact of maltreatment on the overall social and emotional well-being of children who have experienced abuse or neglect. HHS is examining and responding to issues of psychotropic drug use within this context with the goal of building the capacity of child welfare systems to both identify the needs of children and youth who have been maltreated and deliver effective, evidence-based interventions to meet those needs. Certainly this includes strengthened protocols for the prescription and monitoring of psychotropic medications; more broadly, though, it requires that child welfare systems have increased ability to deliver effective psychosocial interventions, such as Trauma-Focused Cognitive-Behavioral Therapy, as treatment strategies alone or, when appropriate, in conjunction with pharmaceutical treatments to improve the well-being of the children and youth that they serve. Such a focus on social and emotional well-being increases the likelihood that children who enter foster care exit to reunification, guardianship, or adoption sooner and better equipped to become healthy, contributing adults.

When I became the director of the Illinois Department of Child and Families Services (DCFS) in 2003, the state had seen a dramatic reduction in the number of children in the foster care system. However, our data indicated that the children who were in the state's custody exhibited significant emotional and behavioral problems. There was no question as to the need for intervention and treatment to address the complex needs resulting from the maltreatment these children had experienced. At the same time, biological, foster, and adoptive parents shared with me the concerns that they had with regard to the psychotropic medications with which their children were treated. Many felt that these drugs were being overprescribed and were causing adverse side-effects, such a sedation, weight gain, and attention problems. A common sentiment among these parents was that they lacked the expertise to make decisions about psychotropic medications or monitor their use and side-effects in their children. Their concerns were representative of the lack of capacity in the child welfare system to understand and oversee pharmacological treatment of children's behavioral and psychological issues. During my tenure as director, DCFS developed a comprehensive system of protocols and safeties to ensure that psychotropic medications are prescribed responsibly and monitored consistently. This included:

- requiring that all prescriptions be reviewed and approved at the state Deputy Director level;
- establishing time-limits for reviews to ensure that necessary treatment was not delayed;
- developing an electronic database for tracking all prescriptions for children in foster care;
- creating "red flags" in the database that elevated certain cases, such as those in which three or more medications were prescribed, for more thorough review; and
- establishing best practice guidelines and distributing them to prescribers. The electronic database was also designed to identify providers whose patterns of prescribing differed from the guidelines.

The net result of these activities was greater longitudinal oversight of the pharmacological treatment of young people in foster care. We collected better data on how psychotropic medications were being used among this population, and important safety checks were established to ensure that use was appropriate and responsible.

OVERVIEW

Over the last decade and a half, the child welfare system has become 27 percent smaller, declining from 559,000 children in 1998 to just over 400,000 in 2010.[1] Nearly all states have been able to reduce the number of children in foster care significantly by providing necessary support services to families to prevent children from coming into care, and, when they do come into care, moving them more quickly to permanent placements, such as reunification, guardianship, or adoption. However, as the system continues to decrease in size, the children who have remained in foster care are more likely to have emotional and behavioral problems that hinder healthy functioning and make it difficult to achieve permanency. Children who experience the trauma of maltreatment have complex needs and require a comprehensive set of services to overcome the social and emotional impact of abuse and neglect to be successful in life. As the child welfare system continues to reduce in size, it must concurrently build the capacity to identify the repercussions of maltreatment and deliver effective interventions that facilitate healing and recovery.

Social-emotional, behavioral, and mental health needs of children in child welfare

Children who come to the attention of the child welfare system have disproportionally high rates of social-emotional, behavioral, and mental health challenges. When examining rates of mental health diagnoses or behavior problems requiring clinical intervention, it becomes clear that the impacts of abuse and neglect on child and adolescent functioning are profound. A key source of information about the social and emotional well-being of and use of psychotropic medications with children who have experienced maltreatment comes from the *National Survey of Child and Adolescent Well-Being* (NSCAW), a longitudinal study required by the Personal Responsibility and Work Opportunity Reconciliation Act of 1996 and overseen by the Administration on Children and Families. NSCAW has been the source of invaluable information about how children who have been maltreated are doing over time and across domains – in school, at home, as they receive services, and as they become adults. Although it provides high-quality data that directly informs the work of child welfare and mental health providers, the continuation of this important survey is at risk. Without ongoing funding from Congress, we will lose our best window into the lives of children who experience maltreatment.

NSCAW and other sources of information about the well-being of children and youth known to child welfare demonstrate the impact of maltreatment on social-emotional, behavioral and mental health:

- 23 percent of children 17 and under who have experienced maltreatment have behavior problems requiring clinical intervention. Clinical-level behavior problems are almost three times as common among this population as among the general population.[2]

- 35 percent of children 17 and under who have experienced maltreatment demonstrate clinical-level problems with social skills – more than twice the rate of the general population.[3]
- Both internalizing problems (e.g., depression, anxiety, being withdrawn) and externalizing problems (e.g., aggression, delinquency) are common in children who have experienced maltreatment. Among children who enter foster care, approximately one third have clinical-level behavior problems.[4]
- Children in foster care are more likely to have a mental health diagnosis than other children. In a study of foster youth between the ages of 14 and 17, 63 percent met the criteria for at least one mental health diagnosis at some point in their life. The most common were Oppositional Defiant Disorder/Conduct Disorder, Major Depressive Disorder/Major Depressive Episode, Attention Deficit/Hyperactivity Disorder, and Posttraumatic Stress Disorder.[5]
- By the time they are 17, 62 percent of youth in foster care will exhibit both symptoms of mental health disorder and symptoms of trauma.[6]
- Although they make up only three percent of the Medicaid population under age 18, children in foster care account for 32 percent of the recipients of behavioral health services in this group.[7]

Psychotropic medication use among children in foster care

According to a 2010 study, children in 13 states who are in foster care and enrolled in Medicaid were prescribed antipsychotic medications at nearly nine times the rate of children enrolled in Medicaid who were not in foster care.[8] Over three years, 22 percent of children in foster care will have taken a psychotropic drug at some point.[9] Although numerous studies have demonstrated that rates of psychotropic medication prescription are high among this group, it is unclear to what extent these rates may be reflecting, at least in part, the increased distress among children who have experienced maltreatment, though other factors may also be playing a role.

Studies have shown the following, with regard to the prevalence of psychotropic drug use and factors influencing the likelihood of use among children in foster care:

- *Age*: Children in foster care are more likely to be prescribed psychotropics as they grow older, with 3.6 percent of 2-5 year-olds taking medication at a given time, 16.4 percent of 6-11 year-olds, and 21.6 percent of 12-16 year-olds. The likelihood that a child will be prescribed multiple psychotropic medications also increases with age.[10]

- *Gender*: Males in foster care are more likely to be receiving psychotropic medications (19.6 percent) than their female counterparts (7.7 percent).[11]
- *Behavioral Concerns*: Children scoring in the clinical range on the Child Behavioral Checklist, a common tool for assessing both internalizing and externalizing behavioral issues among children and youth, are much more likely than those with subclinical scores to receive psychotropic medications.[12]

Additionally, researchers have identified some patterns of prescription of psychotropic medication to children in foster care that may be problematic:

- Documented geographic variation in psychotropic medication use among children coming into contact with child welfare indicates that factors other than clinical need impact prescription. One study found that children in Texas were five times as likely as children in California to be taking psychotropic drugs. The varying rates of use cannot be attributed to population differences, suggesting that factors other than clinical need, such as gender and age, may be influencing the practice of prescribing psychotropic medications.[13]
- To treat the multiple mental and behavioral health symptoms that a child may exhibit, more than one drug–and often more than one type of medication–are prescribed. Among children in foster care taking psychotropic medication, 21.3 percent are receiving monotherapy (one class of psychotropic medication), 41.3 percent are taking three or more classes of psychotropics, 15.4 percent are taking medication from four or more classes, and 2.1 percent taking five or more classes of drugs.[14] Although children with histories of maltreatment often present with complex, co-morbid conditions, evidence of the effectiveness of concomitant psychotropic use is scant. There is no research to support the use of five or more psychotropic drugs, yet we know that a small number of children in foster care are receiving medications at these levels. Further, taking multiple medications within and across classes increases the risk of adverse effects, including drug interactions.

It is clear that the current use of psychotropic medications among children, particularly children in foster care, goes beyond that which is supported by empirical research. In the absence of such research, it is not possible to know all of the short- and long-term effects, both positive and negative, of psychotropic medications on young minds.

DEPARTMENTAL ACTIVITIES

The Department of Health and Human Services (HHS) has undertaken an interagency effort to understand the unique needs of children who have experienced abuse or neglect and develop a coordinated strategy to build the capacity of child welfare systems to meet these needs. Research has demonstrated that maltreatment has long-lasting, adverse effects in all domains of development. As our understanding about the multidimensional impact of maltreatment has increased, our knowledge of effective, evidence-based treatments, both psychosocial and pharmacological, has grown as well. However, the child welfare system has lacked the capacity to incorporate this knowledge and consistently apply it to improve the lives of children who have been abused or neglected. Through ongoing, coordinated efforts across the Department to build knowledge and encourage best practices, HHS is working to build the capacity of child welfare, children's mental health, and state Medicaid systems to both recognize the social-emotional, mental, and behavioral health consequences of maltreatment and deliver a mix of services that effectively responds to the complex needs of the children they serve.

To this end, a joint letter from the Administration on Children and Families (ACF), Centers for Medicare & Medicaid Services (CMS) and the Substance Abuse and Mental Health Services Administration (SAMHSA) was sent out on November 23, 2011 to raise awareness of these issues at the state level and to share expanded opportunities that will be offered to strengthen their systems of prescribing and monitoring psychotropic medication use among children in foster care. These opportunities draw on the existing authority and resources of HHS and are part of a collaborative, department-wide strategy to address this issue.

Additionally, a workgroup with representatives from HHS agencies- ACF, CMS, SAMHSA, the Agency for Healthcare Research and Quality (AHRQ), the Food and Drug Administration (FDA) and the National Institutes of Health (NIH) convened in the summer of 2011 with an initial task of examining the monitoring and oversight of psychotropic medications among children in foster care.

As an initial task, the workgroup gathered information about the need for mental and behavioral health services among children in foster care, as well as the use of psychotropic medications in this population. Peer-reviewed journal articles, research reports, reviews of state practices, and conversations with expert researchers and clinicians informed this process. HHS is disseminating this information widely and continues to seek emerging knowledge about the impact of maltreatment and what works to meet the complex needs of children known to the child welfare system. Additionally, HHS is funding demonstration and research projects related to the use of psychotropic medications and/or behavioral interventions for children in foster care.

Much is known about how child welfare systems can deliver more effective services to treat children and youth who have experienced maltreatment. A number of professional organizations have built upon a wealth of empirical and practice-based evidence to create guidelines for the treatment of children known to child welfare, including the prescription and monitoring of psychotropic medications. Several states and jurisdictions have taken steps to both improve controls on psychotropic medications for children in foster care and increase their ability to identify and respond to the consequences of maltreatment. HHS is encouraging child welfare systems to learn about what works and undertake changes to implement best practices based on the existing professional guidelines and state examples, both of which are grounded in rigorous research or prior successful application. This includes the development of guidance and provision of technical assistance to states, territories, and tribes to support the building of capacity to recognize and respond to the needs of children who have been abused or neglected.

Future Actions

HHS has identified concrete actions in the three areas outlined above: (1) increasing oversight and monitoring of psychotropic medications, (2) expanding the evidence base for effectively responding to the needs of maltreated children, and (3) expanding the use of evidence-based screening, diagnosis, and treatment of social-emotional, behavioral, and mental health issues among children who have experienced abuse or neglect.

Expanding oversight and monitoring of psychotropic medications. HHS is strongly committed to the appropriate prescription and use of psychotropic therapies for children. In the coming months, ACF will issue guidance to states on best practices for monitoring psychotropic drug prescriptions for foster children.

State practices regarding prescription and oversight of psychotropic medications vary widely, and experts agree that greater controls are needed to ensure safe and appropriate use. According to the Child and Family Services Improvement and Innovation Act of 2011 (P.L. 112-34), states must develop their own psychotropic medication monitoring procedures and describe them in their Child and Family Services Plans (CFSP). In advance of their 2012 Annual Plan and Services Report (APSR) submission (annual plans update and amend CFSPs, which are completed every five years), HHS will provide technical assistance, including the dissemination of guidelines developed by professional associations and information about exemplary practices in place in some states.

Additional ongoing activities will enhance psychotropic medication oversight. CMS will work with states to enhance their Drug Utilization Review (DUR) programs, which allow states to monitor dispensing at the point-of-sale, the pharmacy counter, and to influence prescriber behavior. CMS also will encourage providers to adopt, implement, upgrade, and meaningfully use Electronic Health Records (EHRs) in order to access the Medicaid and Medicare EHR incentive payments. EHRs can improve the consistency and quality of health services for children, especially those whose residences changes frequently. The development of quality health homes, standards for behavioral health, and behavioral health coverage for children and adults are among the practices that CMS will promote.

Expanding the evidence base. Efforts to expand the evidence base regarding the needs of children who have been maltreated are twofold. First, HHS is actively disseminating existing information about effective treatment of children known to child welfare, including the prescription and monitoring of psychotropic medications. Among other resources, this includes a report funded by AHRQ summarizing the findings of a 16-state consortium of state Medicaid medical directors developing best practices to improve the use of antipsychotic medications in children in Medicaid. Mechanisms for disseminating this and additional information about psychotropic medications and behavioral interventions for children in foster care include webinars; a joint letter to state child welfare, Medicaid, and mental health directors from ACF, CMS, and SAMHSA; an Information Memorandum and subsequent Program Instruction to child welfare directors; and a compilation of resources on the

Child Welfare Information Gateway, an online clearinghouse of materials for child welfare and related professionals.

Second, HHS is growing the evidence base by funding research and demonstration projects that investigate both client-level interventions and system strategies to improve well-being outcomes for children and families. AHRQ has contracted for an evidence review of interventions that address child exposure to familial trauma in the form of maltreatment or family violence. Meanwhile, the Administration on Children, Youth and Families (ACYF) has organized its discretionary funding to promote the social and emotional well-being of children and youth who have experienced maltreatment. For example, in FY 2011, a cluster of five grantees received a total of $3.2 million to implement evidence-based, trauma-focused practices and evaluate their impact on safety, permanency, and well-being outcomes. Findings from research and demonstration projects supported by HHS will also be widely disseminated to a variety of stakeholders.

Increasing the use of evidence-based screening, diagnosis, and treatment. Other HHS actions will serve to expand the use of evidence-based and best practices for the identification and treatment of social-emotional, behavioral, and mental health problems among children who have experienced maltreatment. HHS supports the use of evidence-based interventions by disseminating information about what works (for instance, via the National Registry of Evidence-Based Programs and Practices and the National Child Traumatic Stress Network) and providing funding for implementation of strategies grounded in rigorous research (e.g., Maternal, Infant and Early Childhood Home Visiting Program). These practices serve to identify and assess the needs of children who are suffering from the negative effects of abuse and neglect, and to target and deliver the appropriate services to meet children's identified needs. As child welfare systems build the capacity to recognize the consequences of maltreatment with greater precision, their delivery of services will be more tailored, and therefore more effective and efficient.

Because children in foster care are involved with multiple systems, including education, health, mental health, Medicaid, and others, a coordinated, multi-system approach is necessary to meaningfully improve outcomes for this population. HHS is working to facilitate state-level collaborations for the purposes of fostering improved behavioral health diagnosis, treatment, and tracking of all children, including those in foster care. In addition to holding joint webinars and disseminating materials across systems, ACYF, CMS, and SAMHSA will, in July 2012, convene state child welfare, Medicaid, and mental health directors to develop action plans for enhancing oversight of psychotropic medications and improving well-being for children in foster care.

It should be noted that increasing the capacity of child welfare systems to conduct evidence- based screening, assessment, and treatment requires enhancing the clinical competencies of the workforce. As the research I have shared demonstrates, children who have experienced maltreatment have a complex behavioral profile requiring specialized services. In order to deliver these services, which we know can be effective, it is necessary to build the capacity of the child welfare workforce to recognize and respond to the impacts of abuse and neglect.

CONCLUSION

The research tells us that most of the children in foster care receiving psychotropic medications have legitimate needs that require careful, comprehensive intervention. There are effective treatments for the mental health disorders and trauma symptoms common among children known to child welfare, and efforts undertaken to ensure the appropriate use of psycho-tropics for these children must be accompanied by increased availability of evidence-based psychosocial treatments that meet the complex needs of children who have experienced maltreatment.

The experience of maltreatment can derail the development of a child and severely hinder his or her chances for success throughout life. However, we know that some children who have been abused or neglected do not develop the myriad problems listed above. That tells us that although children who have been maltreated face immense challenges, they are incredibly resilient. We also know that even among children who do develop social-emotional, behavioral, and mental health problems, healing and recovery are possible. With the right tools and capacity, child welfare systems can identify the complex needs of children who have experienced maltreatment and deliver targeted, evidence-based services that help young people overcome the social and emotional impact of abuse and neglect. By addressing these needs, we increase the likelihood that children in foster care will exit to positive, permanent settings, with the skills and resources they need to be successful in life. HHS is working to build the child welfare system's capacity to identify and treat the needs of maltreated children by expanding the evidence base around social- emotional well-being for children in foster care; improving oversight and monitoring of psychotropic medications among this group; and expanding the use of evidence-based screening, assessment, and treatment to promote healing, recovery, and well-being for these children.

Thank you. I look forward to working with you on these issues, and I am happy to take your questions.

Risk of Social-Emotional Problems and Use of Psychotropic Medication, by Placement Setting

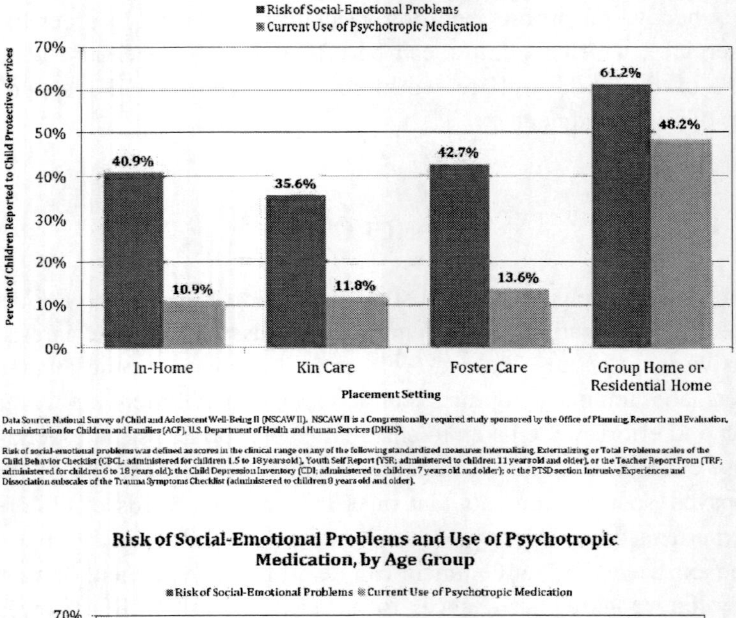

Data Source: National Survey of Child and Adolescent Well-Being II (NSCAW II). NSCAW II is a Congressionally required study sponsored by the Office of Planning, Research and Evaluation, Administration for Children and Families (ACF), U.S. Department of Health and Human Services (DHHS).

Risk of social-emotional problems was defined as scores in the clinical range on any of the following standardized measures: Internalizing, Externalizing or Total Problems scales of the Child Behavior Checklist (CBCL: administered for children 1.5 to 18 years old), Youth Self Report (YSR; administered to children 11 years old and older), or the Teacher Report From (TRF; administered for children 6 to 18 years old); the Child Depression Inventory (CDI; administered to children 7 years old and older); or the PTSD section Intrusive Experiences and Dissociation subscales of the Trauma Symptoms Checklist (administered to children 8 years old and older).

Risk of Social-Emotional Problems and Use of Psychotropic Medication, by Age Group

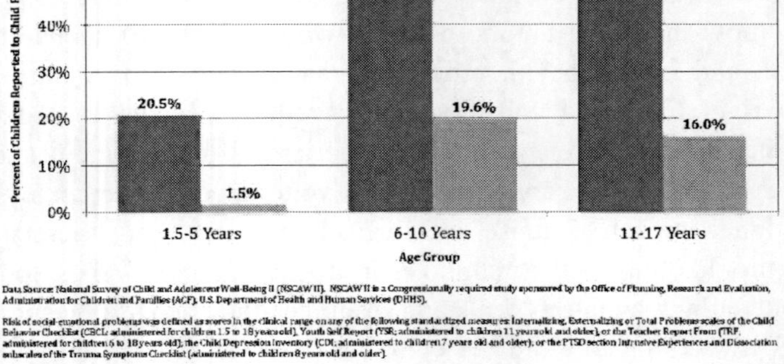

Data Source: National Survey of Child and Adolescent Well-Being II (NSCAW II). NSCAW II is a Congressionally required study sponsored by the Office of Planning, Research and Evaluation, Administration for Children and Families (ACF), U.S. Department of Health and Human Services (DHHS).

Risk of social-emotional problems was defined as scores in the clinical range on any of the following standardized measures: Internalizing, Externalizing or Total Problems scales of the Child Behavior Checklist (CBCL: administered for children 1.5 to 18 years old), Youth Self Report (YSR; administered to children 11 years old and older), or the Teacher Report From (TRF; administered for children 6 to 18 years old); the Child Depression Inventory (CDI; administered to children 7 years old and older); or the PTSD section Intrusive Experiences and Dissociation subscales of the Trauma Symptoms Checklist (administered to children 8 years old and older).

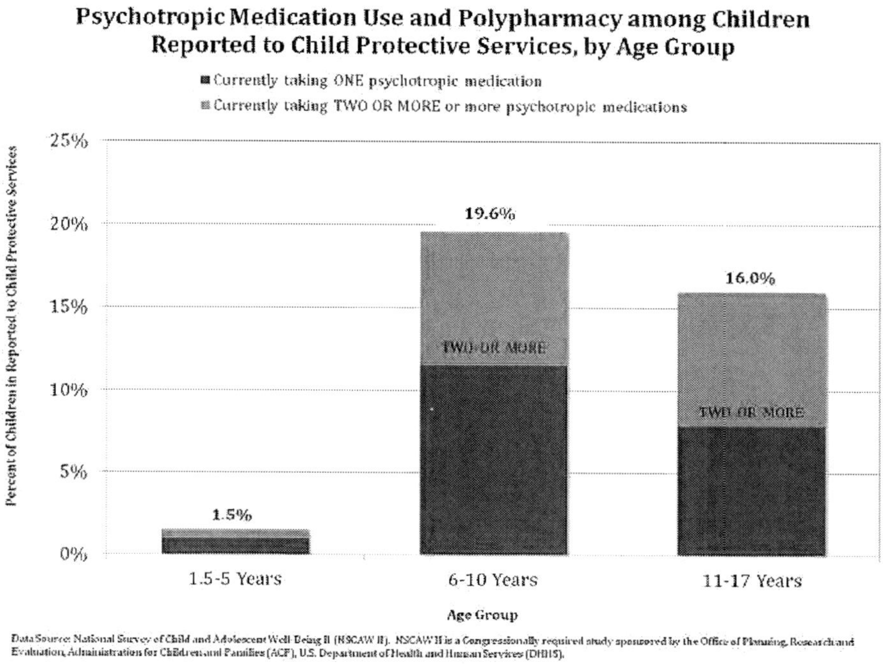

End Notes

[1] Administration for Children and Families (1998-20 10). Adoption and Foster Care Analysis and Reporting System, Reports 11- 18. Washington, DC: US Department of Health and Human Services.

[2] Data source: National Survey for Child and Adolescent Well-Being II

[3] Ibid.

[4] Ibid.

[5] White, CR; Havalchak, A; Jackson, L; O'Brien, K; & Pecora, PJ. (2007). Mental Health, Ethnicity, Sexuality, and Spirituality among Youth in Foster Care: Findings from The Casey Field Office Mental Health Study. Casey Family Programs.

[6] Griffin, G; McClelland, Holzberg, M; Stolbach, B; Maj, N; & Kisiel, C (In Press). Addressing the impact of trauma before diagnosing mental illness in child welfare. *Child Welfare.*

[7] Center for Health Care Strategies, Inc. (Forthcoming). Analysis of Medicaid Claims Data for 2005.

[8] Crystal, S; Olfson, M; Huang, C; Pincus, H; & Gerhard, T. (2009). Broadened use of atypical antipsychotics: Safety, effectiveness, and policy challenges. *Health Affairs.* 28(5):770. (http://content.healthaffairs.org/content/28/5/w770.full.html)

[9] Leslie, LK; Raghavan, R; Zhang, J; & Aarons, GA. (2010). Rates of psychotropic medication use over time among youth in child welfare/child protective services. *Journal of Child and Adolescent Psychopharmacology.* 20(2): 135.

[10] Raghavan, R; Zima, BT; Anderson, RM; Leibowitz, AA; Schuster, MA; & Landsverk, J. (2005). Psychotropic medication use in a national probability sample of children in the child welfare system. *Journal of child and adolescent psychopharmacology*. 15(1):97.

[11] Ibid.

[12] Ibid.

[13] Raghavan, R; Gyanesh, L; Kohl, P; & Hamilton, B. (2010). Interstate variations in psychotropic medication use among a national sample of children in the child welfare system. *Child Maltreatment.* 15(2): 121-131.

[14] Zito, JM; et al. (2008). Psychotropic medication patterns among youth in foster care. *Pediatrics*. 121(1): e157.

In: Medicating Foster Care Children... ISBN: 978-1- 61942-889-8
Editors: R. L. Ray and M. A. Watkins

Chapter 4

MEDICATING FOSTER CHILDREN HEARING-SALO TESTIMONY*

Matt Salo

Good morning Chairman Carper, Ranking Member Brown, and distinguished members of the committee. My name is Matt Salo, and I am the Executive Director of the National Association of Medicaid Directors (NAMD). We appreciate the opportunity to testify before you today on an issue of critical importance in our health care system.

MEDICAID

Medicaid is the nation's health care safety net. Jointly financed by the states and the federal government, Medicaid will spend more than $400 billion this year to provide health care to more than 60 million Americans. The program is administered by the states within a broad federal framework which leads to enormous variation across states in terms of who is covered, what services are provided, and how those services are delivered and paid for. Furthermore, within any given state, Medicaid's role is broad, varied, and

* This is an edited, reformatted and augmented version of the statement of Matt Salo, Executive Director, National Association of Medicaid Directors, before the Committee on Homeland Security and Governmental Affairs, Hearing on "The Financial and Societal Costs of Medicating America's Foster Children."

complex. Medicaid funds more than 40 percent of all births, and the majority of all publicly financed long-term care in this country. It also provides most of the nation's funding for HIV/AIDS-related treatments, mental health services, and others. It is therefore very difficult to talk simplistically about Medicaid (either nationally, or within a state), despite its incredible importance in the U.S. health care system.

NAMD is a newly formed organization created with the sole purpose of providing a home for the nation's Medicaid directors and we represent all 56 of the state, territorial and DC agency heads. Our two broad objectives are to give the Medicaid directors a strong, unified voice on national and federal matters as well as helping develop a robust body of technical assistance and best practices for them to improve their own programs. While no two programs look exactly alike, the directors are unified in their heartfelt desire to improve the health and health care of the growing number of Americans who rely on the program.

Pharmaceutical Coverage for Children in Foster Care

Pharmaceutical coverage and expenditures have been a large and growing concern of the Medicaid directors for a number of years. Psychotropics pose a unique concern primarily because the trends in costs and utilization are far outstripping every other baseline. Careful analysis of the data implies that this is a result of many factors, some legitimate, others less so. Concerns include both overutilization and inappropriate utilization, and this is true for adults, seniors, and, unfortunately, children as well.

As noted in the GAO report, this is also true, and especially concerning for one particularly vulnerable population, children in foster care. While psychotropic medications show enormous promise in treating a wide variety of serious conditions, there are clearly concerns about how current prescribing patterns can negatively impact the foster care population. The GAO report pointed out serious potential problems in three primary areas: the concomitant use of five or more psychotropics; prescribing doses higher than the maximum levels cited by FDA guidelines; and the prescribing of psychotropics to infants under 1 year old.

There is no question that subjecting our most vulnerable citizens to bad medicine is unacceptable and that we can and should and will do better by them.

But there is also no question that this problem is the result of a range of serious flaws in the U.S. health care system: from the prescribing patterns of physicians to the lack of oversight of a variety of levels of government, the lack of effectively promulgated health information technology, and the fragmented nature of the relationship between acute care and behavioral health in this country. As such, solutions will require coordinated efforts from states, the federal government, mental health professionals, primary care practitioners, researchers, and others.

By definition, children in foster care are covered primarily by Medicaid, and, as noted in the report, "they tend to have more numerous and serious medical and mental health conditions than do other children." While this does not excuse the delivery of substandard care, it does help to explain why psychotropic prescribing patterns for this population are higher than for the general population. We also note a recent study in the medical journal *Pediatrics* that shows that psychotropic prescribing patterns for children in foster care are even higher than those in the SSI population, who are by definition facing much more serious disabilities than the general population. This is likely true because many of the children who qualify for SSI do so because of physical, as opposed to behavioral/mental disabilities. To that extent, the foster care population may legitimately require more significant behavioral intervention than the overall SSI population.

There are other reasons to make sure we are making valid comparisons before drawing conclusions. In conversations with the medical and behavioral health experts in the states surveyed for the report, questions that warrant exploration were raised about the survey. For example, multiple prescriptions might reflect a prescriber legitimately cycling through a variety of potential medications in order to find the one that works best for an individual. Similarly, there are instances where multiple psychotropics may well be in the best medical and behavioral needs of a given individual. Further analysis of prescribing patterns for infants show that many examples are for Benadryl. This is not to excuse unacceptable behavior, or rationalize away serious problems where they exist, simply that more analysis is needed to figure out the nature and scope of the real underlying problems.

CHALLENGES

There are unfortunately a number of reasons why state oversight policy, or medical practice may have failed to keep up with the ever changing literature or other developments. These are not meant to be excuses for failure to act, but indicative of the breadth of the challenges that face systemic reform. Furthermore, it cannot be stressed enough how unique are the challenges faced by the children in the foster care system.

While government has an obligation to lead, doing so in violation of clear community opposition is fraught with risk, and pyrrhic victories are often short lived. As states grapple with finding solutions to the epidemic of over- and misuse of psychotropics in general, they often face opposition from the manufacturers of these products, from mental health advocates (who in many cases are funded in large part by these same manufacturers), and from the community at large, who tend to resist government intrusion into a doctor-patient relationship often viewed as sacrosanct.

In some states, this has resulted in state legislative action that has placed absolute prohibitions on prior authorization of psychotropics like atypical antipsychotics. These laws place significant barriers on state pharmacy managers in their efforts to ensure compliance with the latest practice guidelines. While state legislative barriers are not permanently set in stone, resolving them does require different strategies than in addressing state-level executive branch policy.

These challenges also play out in the complicated relationship between state foster care workers, the children in the system, and the prescribers themselves. A lot of behavioral problems in foster care kids are as a result of trauma which is under-diagnosed and requires specialized treatment approaches.

As a practical matter, in an emergency, most prescribers are more likely to add medications than discontinue them, and effectively minimizing medication use requires a stable ongoing treatment relationship with a prescriber – a relationship that is rare, especially among older children who can change placements frequently, seeing a different prescriber each time.

State agencies also face challenges in recruiting and retaining sufficiently trained staff who possess the clinical expertise necessary to challenge a prescriber's recommendation to treat with psychotropics. One state in particular had to abandon an attempt to strengthen the hand of foster care workers in these situations, when it became clear that BA/BS or MSW educated workers would face significant liability issues when disagreeing with prescribers.

SOLUTIONS

In the short term, I would note that in my conversations with the states that were a part of the GAO study, all were undertaking efforts to address the identified shortcomings. I know that your staff have had extensive conversations with many, if not all, of these states, but we would be happy to continue to work with you if there is any further outstanding follow up required.

But above and beyond these individual efforts, there is also a need for broader systemic reform. There are a number of solutions that can and should be implemented to help improve this situation. 1) The GAO report recommends promulgating additional federal guidance from HHS to the states; 2) More clinical research is needed on the effects and implications of treating children of any age and in any situation with psychotropics that have only been tested on adults; 3) More work needs to be done to break down the barriers to coordinating and integrating care for vulnerable populations in Medicaid, with an added focus on the varied, complex and challenging behavioral health conditions experienced by children in foster care; 4) While Medicaid coverage and payment policy can and should change, many of the challenges in this issue are medical policy issues, and as such, require the broader medical community to also adapt; and 5) NAMD, working collaboratively with key partners such as the Medicaid medical directors and the state mental health program directors can develop and disseminate best practices in this area and work with states to implement them;

More HHS Guidance

While HHS has provided some guidance thus far, states would clearly welcome additional information. On behalf of our members, NAMD is committed to working with HHS, across the various agencies that impact this population, including the Administration on Children and Families (ACF) the Substance Abuse and Mental Health Services Administration (SAMHSA), the Center for Medicaid and CHIP Services (CMCS), and others. This is especially true in instances where state Medicaid agency policymakers need additional tools or leverage to convince policymakers in the state legislative branch or even state medical association leadership about changes to current policy.

The American Academy of Child and Adolescent Psychiatry (AACAP) guidelines contain four broad categories: consent, oversight, consultation, and information sharing. The preliminary investigation into the six sample states demonstrates a wide range of compliance with the non-binding recommendations in these four categories. We know that HHS is developing comprehensive guidance, and combining those recommendations with the power of transparency on this poorly-studied issue should help states improve their practices and improve the lives of foster children entrusted to our care.

Research on Psychotropic Impacts on Children

There are three major holes in the body of medical research relevant to this situation. The broadest is that there is not enough evidence on the comparative effectiveness of the various generations of psychotropics. FDA's mandate is to approve new pharmaceuticals based on performance relative to placebos, not relative to existing products.

A second relevant issue is the lack of understanding of how psychotropic drugs affect children in general. Children generally do not participate in FDA clinical trials for a variety of reasons, but there must be ways to work around this barrier to better understand how these powerful substances affect developing minds.

Finally, as noted in the GAO report, in an unspecified state, "57 percent of foster children were diagnosed with a mental disorder – nearly 15 times that of nonfoster children receiving Medicaid assistance." However, the report goes on to say that "very little research has been done on the use of psychotropic drugs in foster children with severe symptoms. This limits the information available to providers on how best to treat their conditions." The challenges faced by children that result in their placement in foster care combined with the challenges they face once in the system are nothing like those faced by either children in the general population, or even non-foster care children diagnosed with several mental illness. More work is needed to evaluate these unique challenges and to prepare for them.

Integrated and Coordinated Care

Care coordination— the alignment of treatments, various health professionals and regular care givers around a care plan for individuals with mental and physical health problems—is essential to good health outcomes and too often lacking in our nation's health care system. Further complicating good care, is the fragmentation between the fields of mental and physical health care. Privacy concerns, divergent professional training, and splintered payment and coverage systems are just a few of the reasons why behavioral and physical health needs are thought of and addressed separately.

As noted in the GAO report, "foster children who change placements often do not have a consistent caretaker to plan treatment, offer consent, and provide oversight...changes in placement pose significant challenges for agencies, foster parents, and providers with regard to providing continuity of health care services and maintaining uninterrupted information on children's medical needs and courses of treatment." For them, the fragmentation between mental health and primary care is exacerbated by the transitory nature of their care and treatment regimen.

Medicaid, Medicare and private payers are actively investing in care coordination efforts, including medical homes, health IT and evidence-based medicine. These efforts should benefit foster children, but they are likely insufficient to address the range of problems without focused initiatives.

Medical Policy Changes

As stated by the AACAP, "the ultimate judgment regarding the care of a particular patient must be made by the clinician in light of all of the circumstances presented by the patient and his or her family, the diagnostic and treatment options available, and available resources." Without disputing that assessment, it is clear that clinicians desperately need more information about not only the options available, but better data and analysis to determine their effectiveness and consequences. However, it is not enough to simply assume that more research will lead automatically and quickly to significant changes in practice. It is the medical professionals themselves, aided by their trade associations that must similarly commit to reforming how they practice medicine.

NAMD Best Practices

As I mentioned earlier, one of the two primary functions of our association is to help identify and disseminate best practices across all states.

In this particular area, we have been and will continue to be strongly supportive of the efforts of groups like the Medicaid Medical Directors Learning Network (MMDLN) and the National Association of State Mental Health Program Directors (NASMHPD) to work with states to address these challenges. They have formed a consortium of 16 states representing about 12 million children and adolescents covered by Medicaid. Their work to date includes: analyses of each state's antipsychotic medical use rates and trends for children, adolescents and those in foster care; the development of a set of safety, quality, or appropriate-use indicators to monitor treatment patterns; identification of state-specific programs and policies that could improve the use of antipsychotic medications; providing a forum for discussion of policies and programs for optimizing antipsychotic medication; and the development of a compendium of state practices that could be shared with other states to address issues related to antipsychotic use in children and adolescents.

This work resides on a public website and is already changing statewide practices across the country. With these tools states have the ability to work with prescribers to provide safer and more effective medication management across Medicaid or any population that chooses to use the guidelines.

In: Medicating Foster Care Children... ISBN: 978-1- 61942-889-8
Editors: R. L. Ray and M. A. Watkins

Chapter 5

MEDICATING FOSTER CHILDREN HEARING-MCCLELLAN TESTIMONY*

Jon McClellan

Mr. Chairman and members of the subcommittee; thank you for inviting me to participate in this important discussion regarding the use of psychotropic medications in foster children.

I am a child psychiatrist at Seattle Children's Hospital, a professor at the University of Washington, and the medical director of Child Study and Treatment Center, the State psychiatric hospital for youth in Washington State.

The high risk practices identified by the GAO study raise significant concerns regarding the treatment of severely mentally ill and vulnerable youth. Although the focus of this study is on foster care, the concerns raised are relevant to all children and adolescents prescribed psychotropic drugs.

Children in foster care often have emotional and behavioral difficulties. The high rate of medication use in this population is not a new discovery, nor does the use of these drugs always imply bad practice. Several psychiatric medications have been studied and approved for use in children and adolescents. When prescribed correctly, these treatments can help reduce suffering and enhance the functioning of young people.

---

* This is an edited, reformatted and augmented version of the statement of Dr. Jon McClellan, Professor, University of Washington, Seattle, Washington, before the Committee on Homeland Security and Governmental Affairs, Hearing on "The Financial and Societal Costs of Medicating America's Foster Children."

However, it is also well documented that many children in the child welfare system do not receive high quality psychiatric services. Treatment too often occurs during times of crisis, without adequate support or access to skilled clinicians and programs capable of providing effective social and behavioral interventions.

In these situations, medications become stopgaps, used to prevent the child from hurting themselves or others, or to help control disruptive behaviors that threaten the child's foster placement. The lack of effective long-term treatment exacerbates the risk for excessive and inappropriate medication use.

This problem is evident in the patterns of high-risk prescriptions identified by the GAO study. As a group, children in foster care were more likely than other children to be treated with multiple psychiatric drugs, and also were more likely to be treated with dosages that exceed recommended standards of care.

These practices impacted thousands of children. Some young people were prescribed as many as 10 different psychotropic drugs at the same time. Some children younger than 5 years of age were prescribed as many as 5 different medicines concurrently.

Unfortunately, such practices are not uncommon. At my state hospital, kids are often admitted taking four or more medications. A few years ago, one young boy admitted to Seattle Children's Hospital was taking 13 different psychotropic drugs. There is no research that justifies these practices.

The most troubling finding of the GAO study is the use of psychotropic drugs in infants. Most of the prescriptions in babies were for antihistamines, some of which may have been used to treat other types of medical problems. Regardless, there is little research supporting the use of these medicines in very young children, and the prescriptions are concerning.

Furthermore, dozens of babies were prescribed antipsychotics, antidepressants, clonidine or lithium. Some infants were prescribed more than one drug. The use of psychotropic medications in babies defies both standard of care and common sense.

The findings of the GAO study strongly suggest the need for better oversight. The Best Principals outlined by the American Academy of Child and Adolescent Psychiatry provide a useful set of monitoring guidelines.

Washington State has implemented a model system to oversee psychotropic drugs. Criteria were developed to identify prescriptions that exceed safety thresholds, based on dose, number of medications or age of the child. For prescriptions flagged by this process, a second opinion by a child psychiatrist is required before the medication is dispensed. This oversight system has reduced high-risk prescriptions, and over a two-year period, saved the State 1.2 million dollars.

The results of the GAO study also strongly call for more research. A hodgepodge of prescribing practices occurs in part because none of our current treatments work well enough. Genetics and neurobiological sciences have advanced substantially over the past decade, in large part due to the leadership of the National Institute of Mental Health. Nonetheless, given the marked complexity of brain functioning, the underlying causes of most psychiatric illnesses remain unknown. Without known causes, research on intervention inevitably struggles. We need continued investment, both fiscal and intellectual, in order to develop safer and more effective treatments, and to eventually find cures.

Thank you for listening.

INDEX

Y

Z